HOW TO EAT

A New Proactive Diet Approach for a Better Life

HOW TO EAT

A New Proactive Diet Approach for a Better Life

Bin Ke

COPYRIGHT © 2012 BY INTERNATIONAL UNITED BUSINESS, INC.

LIBRARY OF CONGRESS CONTROL NUMBER: 2012922515

ISBN:	HARDCOVER	978-1-4797-5791-6
	SOFTCOVER	978-1-4797-5790-9
	EBOOK	978-1-4797-5792-3

All rights reserved. No part of this book may be reproduced or transmitted in any form or by any means, electronic or mechanical, including photocopying, recording, or by any information storage and retrieval system, without permission in writing from the copyright owner.

This book offers a new **comprehensive how-to-eat guide** that has taken into consideration foods, habits, and biology factors. The book provides unique effective strategies to help individuals achieve advanced level of eating and life-long healthy weight.

This book was printed in the United States of America.

To order additional copies of this book, contact:
Xlibris Corporation
1-888-795-4274
www.Xlibris.com
Orders@Xlibris.com
125522

Contents

CHAPTER 1 Introduction 1

   1.1 Why Most Diets Don't Work 2

   1.2 Proactive Diet Approach (PDA) 4

   1.3 Comparing PDA with Other Diets 7

   1.4 How to Use the Proactive Diet Approach (PDA) 11

CHAPTER 2 Eat the Best Foods 13

   2.1 Best Vegetable Choices 15

   2.2 Best Fruit Choices 26

   2.3 Best Grains 33

   2.4 Best Protein Foods 38

   2.5 Best Foods in Other Food Groups 44

   2.6 Summary 49

CHAPTER 3 Avoid the Worst Foods 51

   3.1 Most Harmful Foods 53

   3.2 Undesirable Foods 58

   3.3 Summary 62

CHAPTER 4 Achieve Life-Long Healthy Weight 65

   4.1 Obesity Cancer Risk and Epidemic 65

4.2 Understand the Basics of Weight Loss 66

    4.2.1 It's Your Own Hormones 66

    4.2.2 Ins and Outs of Calories 69

    4.2.3 Know Your Body Mass Index (BMI) 72

4.3 PDA Strategies for Weight Management 73

    4.3.1 How to Reduce In Calories 74

    4.3.2 How to Increase Out Calories 76

    4.3.3 How to Outsmart Your Hormones with Low Glycemic Index (GI) Foods 77

4.4 Summary 80

CHAPTER 5 Choose Organic 83

    5.1 Common Vegetables and Fruits 84

    5.2 Meats and Seafood 86

    5.3 Genetically Modified Foods 88

    5.4 How to Read Organic Labels 89

    5.5 Summary 90

CHAPTER 6 Conclusion 93

    6.1 It's Never Too Late 94

    6.2 Every Choice Has Big Impact 95

    6.3 This Book Makes It Easy for You 96

    6.4 Improve Wellbeing 97

    6.5 Lifelong Healthy Weight 98

APPENDIX A Best Foods for Each Food Group 101
    List of Best Vegetables 101
    List of Best Fruits 103
    List of Best Grains 105
    List of Best Proteins 106
    List of Other Best Foods 108
    List of Best Vegetables Based on Single Nutrient 109

APPENDIX B Worst Foods to Avoid 111
    List of Most Harmful Foods 111
    List of Undesirable Foods 112

APPENDIX C Low Glycemic Index (GI) Foods 113
    Examples of Low GI Foods in Different Food Groups 113

APPENDIX D Glossary 115

APPENDIX E References 121

APPENDIX F Disclaimer 129

CHAPTER 1

Introduction

Eating is no longer as simple as in the time of our ancestors. The choices of foods have definitely become more complex in modern times.

Many people like to improve their diets whether it is because that they'd like to eat healthier, or they are not satisfied with their body weight, or they want to have more energy and feel good, or they'd like to eat well to reduce risk of diseases, or they have high aspirations to live to 100 years old and beyond. But lacking the right information and not knowing where to begin is preventing them from getting the desired result from their efforts.

When people are left on their own to figure out what to eat, many of them are plain wrong or misguided when they make daily decisions about what to eat. Many of them eat to give themselves chronic diseases like cancer, heart disease, and diabetes. We are free to choose what we eat, how much we eat, how to eat, and our belief about food for whatever reasons. But we could not choose the consequences of what we eat to our body.

The amount of information about what people should eat is overwhelming and there are hundreds of diet plans promoted by researchers, nutritionists, organizations, governments, and commercial entities. They provide people with some useful information and guidance. However, sorting through all the information about foods have become more and more difficult due to the fact that the amount of information is overwhelming, hard to grasp by average people, and sometime the advices from experts are contradicting.

Many dieters have tried diet plans or quick-fix programs to lose weight often in a short period of time. By reviewing and analyzing 31 long-term diet studies rigorously, UCLA researchers concluded that over 83% of dieters regained most of the lost weight after two years.[1] Many dieters worked very hard to lose weight and found out that maintaining weight is much more difficult. People are frustrated and dismayed, and obviously these diet plans are not working for them.

1.1 Why Most Diets Don't Work

Our diet habit is the single most important factor that affects hundreds of moments when we make a choice for food each week. Just like we are driven by habits in many other behaviors in our life, human beings are simply incapable of switching to a very different habit just by knowing that the new habit is supposed to be so good and the old habit is supposed to be bad.

The main reason that most diet plans do not work, are hard to follow, and people are frustrated following them is because most plans believe that improving diets is just about food and the benefits of nutrients without the consideration of habits and biology factors that are equally important in daily food choices.

Adopting a new diet program is a major disruption both biologically and psychologically for dieters, when they suddenly have to eat many new and unfamiliar foods in their daily diet and have to give up many familiar foods that they are used to eating for years. Dieters have to move beyond their comfort zone to start to shop for new foods, learn how to cook them, adjust to the new tastes, and count calories or measure portion sizes. Some dieters are also asked to restrict certain types of foods and nutrients over the long term. *The kind of sudden change is very unnatural to the body, and switching from the existing habits is hard to sustain for most dieters.*

In fact, many people give up on these plans. Human beings, from the young to the old, very few are programmed to be able to do something they know are right or not to do something knowing that it is harmful.

One most important reason why managing weight is so hard and the weight-loss efforts of many people more often failed than succeeded is that they were fighting their own biology.

Leptin is a hormone that regulates appetite, metabolic rate, and fat storage in our bodies. When the level of leptin is low in the body, it signals the brain that fat storage is low and triggers the body to eat more and slow metabolism to conserve energy. Researchers found that when people lose weight, the leptin level drops dramatically, which in turn increases the urge to eat and creates cravings. It is hard to fight against your own hormone, and only 17% of people are able to maintain their weight loss. The other 83% of people regain most of all the weight that they worked so hard to lose after two years. The biology of our body is against weight loss.

The pleasure hormone dopamine in our brains plays a very big part in our diets and other pleasure behaviors like alcohol addiction, drugs, and sex. Dopamine causes common people complete lack of control facing deserts or certain junk foods. It causes obese people to be prone to gluttony and to keep eating even though their bodies do not need food anymore.[2]

Diet plans that are focusing only on nutritional values of foods without consideration of habits and biology factors disrupt people's rhythms and require tremendous willpower to succeed with this unnatural approach. More often than not, these programs will only drive people to feel dismayed, along with the failure. These approaches provide some useful information and many good advices to dieters, but the long-term success of these diets is still elusive for most dieters.

1.2 Proactive Diet Approach (PDA)

The proactive diet approach (PDA) advocated in this book is a very different how-to-eat paradigm that has taken into consideration foods, habits, and biology factors. PDA is a comprehensive guide to help individuals to understand the key elements of diet and their impact to our body, our weight, our mood, and our behavior.

The proactive diet approach (**PDA**) consists of four easy-to-follow and effective strategies that common people can easily adopt in their own pace to get more out of their eating every day while achieving the highest level of eating and life-long healthy weight in the most efficient way:

- Eat the best foods
- Avoid the worst foods
- Achieve life-long healthy weight
- Choose organic

PDA is based on the latest science about food and nutrition. It focuses on small and gradual changes that lead to eating habits that will stick based on the individual's proactive choices, and it takes into consideration the biology factors in our bodies that play an important role in our every eating choice daily.

What makes PDA truly effective for common people is that it simplifies diet into four clear and flexible strategies that people can easily understand and execute. No matter which strategy you choose to execute fully or partially, you are making positive progress toward the goal of having the healthy diet and wellbeing that you want. Instead of a diet program that dictates what you eat, it is always you who are proactively making every decision by your own preference, on your own pace, and no particular order is required to get the best and complete nutrients for your body and achieve the weight loss for the long term.

Eat the Best Foods—Since you're trying to do the best thing for your body by eating healthy anyway, there is no better way than eating the most nutritious foods.

A healthy diet should consist of eating foods from five major food groups: vegetables, fruits, grains, proteins, and other foods. Other food groups consist of any food that is not considered as vegetables, fruits, grains, or protein but is considered an important element of a healthy diet. Olive oils and chocolates are such examples. Oils from plants or fish are liquid fats that provide unique healthy nutrients.

This book makes choosing what to eat very easy by providing a list of best choices for each major food group. If you choose to start with eating the best foods strategy, you could start adding one or two best foods that you could enjoy but are not yet in your weekly diet. As time goes by, when you truly appreciate the benefits that you get and realize how easy it is, naturally you will include another best food in your diet. Eating the best foods is the most direct and efficient way to improve your diet immediately. When you eat the healthiest foods that give your body the most nutrient benefits, you also leave less room for unhealthy foods.

Avoid the Worst Foods—Researches and scientific facts are very clear that an unhealthy diet is the leading cause of human death. Why would we eat to give ourselves major illnesses like a heart disease, cancer, and diabetes? The smartest way to live free of illnesses is to avoid the most harmful foods, which are linked to diseases and disorders.

The book provides a list of the most harmful foods and a list of the most undesirable foods that people should avoid. If you choose to improve your diet by avoiding the worst foods, you could simply start by picking one of the worst foods that you feel most easy to give up. *Even small changes in your diet will have a significant impact to your overall health*. You will feel healthier over time, and naturally you will be motivated to add one more worst or undesirable food to be eliminated from your diet. Not only will you limit your exposure to the harm from the most unhealthy foods, which would give you diseases or ailments, you also leave more room for healthy foods.

Achieve Life-Long Healthy Weight—Managing a proper weight is the best way to maintain health and reduce the risk of major ailments and various disorders. More than any other lifestyle factors, body fatness is convincingly linked to increased risk of six cancers[3] as well as unhealthy heart conditions, diabetes, and many disorders. Obesity has become an epidemic in the United States in the past several decades, with an astounding 35% of adults being obese and two-thirds being overweight.[4]

PDA offers a unique new paradigm to manage healthy weight. Traditional diet control, which only focuses on the food and nutrition aspects, is not enough, and most dieters regain most of the weight they lost within a few years. This book explains that foods, activities, and biology are the three key factors that strongly influence body weight. How to outsmart the hormones in your body that regulate your appetite and metabolism is essential for a successful weight management. Instead of a diet program that dictates what you eat, PDA lets individual dieters proactively make small and gradual change based on each individual's own circumstance, own preference, and own pace that lead to habits that stick. PDA provides a set of unique strategies to outsmart your own hormones that work against weight loss by increasing craving for foods and lowering metabolism when weight loss occurs.

Choose Organic Foods—Some of the best fruits (like apple, blueberries, and strawberries) and best vegetables (like kale, spinach, and bell pepper) are among the most contaminated with pesticide residues if conventionally grown. Conventional meats that we eat are from animals that have been raised with antibiotics and growth hormones and fed with gene-modified corn and soy with pesticide residues. Most conventional vegetables oils are from genetically modified seeds, and most conventional soybeans and corns are genetically modified.

Choosing organic foods is the only way to limit our exposure to harmful toxins from our food supply and genetically modified foods. Eating organic is essential to achieve the highest level of healthy diet.

1.3 Comparing PDA with Other Diets

Many diet plans only focus on foods and nutrients and fail to show people how to make the right choices. Not taking into consideration human habits and biology factors that play important roles in people's daily choice of foods is the main reason why these plans have not helped people achieve the diet that they have intended to.

The proactive diet approach (**PDA**) is a comprehensive guide based on foods, habits, and biology factors, to help common people understand how our bodies and wellbeing are affected by these factors. It is a complete diet approach that is based on latest science and discovery. It is consistent with the standard for a balanced diet, which is the general recommendation by most nutritionists.

What makes PDA a truly effective approach is that it focuses on providing a feasible path for common people to proactively establish a long-term, sustainable habit that is suitable to their own circumstance and in harmony with the universal law of health. It provides unique set of strategies to show individuals how to eat to get the best nutrients, how to avoid the pitfalls of the current food environment, and how to effectively achieve a life-long healthy weight instead of "yo-yo" dieting.

If there exists a top of a healthy diet pyramid, which represents the healthiest eating, PDA offers the fastest path to get to the top of the healthy diet pyramid, comparing with any other diet approaches.

The U.S. government has made many efforts over decades to guide Americans on how to have a healthy diet. The new MyPlate[5] guideline from USDA for Americans for a healthy diet recommends balanced diets with five groups of foods: vegetables, fruits, protein foods, grains, and dairy. But how to make a healthy diet is still hard for people to follow with this MyPlate paradigm as well as the old food pyramid guideline from USDA.

MyPlate gives a list of 65 vegetables, with the recommendation to eat varieties of them. It treats all vegetables the same. In fact, some vegetables are nutrient all-stars like broccoli, kale and sweet potato, which are rich in vitamins and minerals that are shown to protect against cancers, are anti aging, and boost immunity or lower risk of heart diseases. Some vegetables have much less health benefits. The health effects would be very different for dieters who include more of the best vegetables in their daily diets versus those who eat more vegetables with lower nutrient values.

Instead of treating every food the same with a generalized recommendation, Eating the Best Foods strategy of PDA provides a list of best foods for every major food group so that people could choose the foods among the best in each group, which they could enjoy while getting the most nutritional benefits. Comparing with MyPlate or any other diet plans, there is no doubt that PDA is the most direct and efficient way to improve your diet immediately.

MyPlate also lacks information on what foods to avoid. High intake of saturated fats, trans fat, sodium, and sugar is the major factor causing high blood pressure, raising bad cholesterol and blood glucose, and causing heart diseases and diabetes. In 2012, the World Cancer Research Fund (WCRF)[3] published the most comprehensive and authoritative report on cancer risk, which shows convincing link between eating processed meat and red meat to higher cancer risk. MyPlate does not provide any guidance about the foods to avoid.

Avoiding the Worst Foods strategy of PDA gives a list of the most harmful foods, which could increase the risk of major diseases, as well as a list of the most undesirable foods that are likely to be consumed in large quantities and frequently but lack nutrient values or contain unhealthy ingredients. Dieters could proactively make the decision to choose one food at a time from the lists, which that they could give up most easily from their diets. Comparing with MyPlate or any other diets, there is no doubt that the strategy is another very efficient way offered by PDA to improve your diet.

Many dieters have tried diet plans or quick-fix programs to lose weight often in a short period of time. The fact is that long-term successful weight loss is not what most quick-fix programs can achieve.

PDA offers a unique new paradigm to manage weight. The philosophy of PDA is it lets individual dieters proactively make small and gradual changes to their diet based on their own circumstance, own preference, and own pace that lead to habits and weight loss that would stick with them for life. No matter which strategy individual dieters choose to execute fully or partially, dieters are making positive progress toward the goal of healthy weight. PDA does not cause stress or guilt that is commonly associated with other diet programs. Over time the small changes lead to habits that stick with the dieters, and the approach will truly accomplish what many other diet recommendations had failed to do: successful life-long weight loss.

PDA versus Other Diet Plans

Proactive Diet Approach	Other Diet Plans
• Consists of four flexible strategies. Advocates small changes proactively made by dieters, which lead to long-lasting diet habits that stick.	• Are complicated, are not flexible, and require sudden and big changes that are unnatural to dieters biologically and psychologically.
• Provide effective strategies based on foods, habits, and biology factors.	• Focus solely on foods and nutrients
• Is very likely to succeed. Dieters make small and incremental steps based on their own paces and own preferences.	• Are less likely to succeed. Are hard to grasp because of too much information and even harder to stick with the plan.
• Offers a comprehensive guide to achieve advanced level of eating	• Focus on one specific area, like weight loss, detox or the heart's health.
• Offers strategies to achieve life-long healthy weight or long term weight loss.	• Are just quick-fix for the short term with dismal long-term results.

1.4 How to Use the Proactive Diet Approach (PDA)

Wellbeing is not just about weight loss; it is about the absence of disease, being free of pains, having youthfulness and longevity, and your body being in a state filled with energy and vitality, where you are able to enjoy food and the life to the fullest extent.

The proactive diet approach (**PDA**) provides a true credible choice for common people to succeed with their diet goals because it makes it easy for people to make small changes that have immediate benefits, and the changes will naturally become habits overtime. There are four PDA strategies for dieters to choose from to start their journey to better wellbeing.

- Eat the best foods
- Avoid the worst foods
- Achieve life-long healthy weight
- Choose organic

With your goal set, you can start with adding one best food that you truly enjoy, or you could choose one worst food that is most easy for you to give up, or you could replace one food that you always eat with an organic source. If you are not ready to take on running or physical activities, reducing calorie intake is a good start to lose weight. Make small changes, and you will see the positive impact to your body and how you feel about yourself. When you become comfortable with the change, pick another food to add or avoid.

For example, a person can simply choose to add one best food into his/her regular diet, let's say to eat a handful of walnuts as snack or adding walnuts to breakfast. This very nutrient-dense food has an incredible amount of omega-3 content, which is three times more than salmon. Omega-3 fatty acids are considered essential fatty acids required for our bodies to function normally. It helps to reduce inflammation, boosts the heart's health, and is protective against cancers and other conditions. Eating one hundred grams (3.5 ounces) of walnuts[6] will provide nearly 27% of the daily requirement for fiber, an amazing 171% of the daily recommendation for manganese, 79% for copper, 40% for magnesium, 35% for phosphorus, 21% for zinc, 16% for iron, and 10% for calcium. Walnut is also an excellent source of vitamins. Eating one hundred grams will provide 25% of the daily requirement for folate, 23% for thiamin, and 27% for B6. Minerals and vitamins are essential nutrients for keeping the body functioning and healthy.

Adding one best food like walnut seems like a small change, but the impact is very big. Studies have shown that eating a handful of walnuts regularly will significantly reduce the risk of heart diseases, diabetes, cancer, and other chronic ailments and improve memory and other brain functions. By making just one adjustment and reaping the benefits immediately, it is very likely walnut will gradually become part of the person's weekly diet, and over time, the person would become very unlikely to give it up. Why would anyone stop eating a food that offers so many benefits?

PDA is an approach that is based on an individual's unique need and situation. Unlike many diet plans that dictate what you eat and fit everyone into the same diet formula, PDA lets you make the proactive choice on your own pace to achieve the diet goal that you set. You will be rewarded with immediate benefits no how matter how small the change that you make is. The power of eating the most nutritious foods will help you achieve the advanced level of wellbeing in the most efficient way.

CHAPTER 2

Eat the Best Foods

Regular exercise, healthy eating, good sleep, weight control, healthy relationship, and harmony in the environment are the foundations for staying healthy. These elements are essential to the health of most people.

We are what we eat. More than any other element, what we eat has the most significant and direct impact to our body, our mood, and behavior. Eating is not just about losing weight or because we feel hungry. What we eat is an element that is within our control and could make the biggest positive contribution or be the worst threat to our own health.

We make many small choices about food, snacks, and drinks daily. People who consistently make good decisions about what they eat are considered advanced level in diet. These advanced people enjoy life with vibrant health, higher energy, active mental state, and of course longevity. They are free from various pains and minor discomfort and, more importantly, are less likely to have major diseases like cancer, heart disease, and diabetes.

David Murdock is such a person with advanced level of diet. Born in 1923, 89 years old Murdock lost his mother to cancer when he was a teenager. His mother died at the young age of 41. Murdock also lost his most beloved wife of eighteen years to advanced ovarian cancer. His wife Gabriele, who was a member of President's Committee on the Arts and Humanities, died when she was only 43. Neither his wife nor his mother had a family history of cancer. David Murdock believes that he could have saved the life of his wife and his mother had he known what he knows today[1].

About 90 years old, Murdock lives a robust life, with a clear mind and an energy level higher than people several decades younger. He has the ideal bill of health and the blood pressure of a teenager. He was not sick for even a day, free from cold, flu or any illness for nearly thirty years. The secret to the vibrant life that he is enjoying and his ambition to live to 125 years old is mostly due to two things: eating the healthiest foods and daily exercise.

He definitely knows more about what to eat than anyone else. David Murdock, who is from a modest family from a small town in Ohio, is not famous for how he became a multibillionaire on his own, starting from working on his first job in a gas station. He is most well known for his devotion to wellbeing after the loss of his wife, Gabriele. He believes that she would have been still alive had they eaten differently.

He invested 500 million of his own money to create the world's leading research campus in North Carolina, with some of the most famous scientists and researchers in foods and health, in cooperation with eight universities to work together to study the benefits of foods to health and longevity. The campus has the most cutting-edge equipment, including the most powerful magnet in the world, to look at the most minute level of plant molecules and human cells. Other than the research campus, Murdock also made many donations to promote healthy eating, longevity and promoted nutrition and disease prevention through his Dole Nutrition Institute.

David Murdock did not start his healthy eating routine until his sixties, and he has been doing grocery shopping mostly by himself even though he is one of the richest men in America. The foods that he chooses to eat, which are the key to maintaining his advanced level of diet, are available in the supermarkets that we all go to. The story of David Murdock is that eating the healthiest foods is the best path to living an active, satisfying, and vibrant life, which leads to longevity. Anyone could achieve this advanced level of diet, and it is never too late to start. Eating the best foods is the most effective approach to get the healthiest benefits.

This book makes the choice of best foods easy for people who'd like to elevate their diets to the next level in the most effective way.

Healthy eating should consist of eating foods from all five major food groups: vegetables, fruits, grains, proteins, and other foods. A list of best foods that is based on the most up-to-date and mainstream research in nutrition and health is provided for each major food group.

Daily Allowance Recommended by USDA for Adults

Protein	5-6.5 Ounces
Grains	3-4 Ounces
Fruits	1.5-2 Cups
Vegetables	2-3 Cups

2.1 Best Vegetable Choices

The choices of vegetables have a fundamental impact to your health because not every vegetable has the same disease-fighting effect or nutrient benefits. Sweet potatoes have 32 times the amount of vitamin A while kale has 21 times more vitamin A compared with even an excellent vegetable like broccoli. Vitamin A helps to reduce the risk of heart disease and cancer and helps to maintain healthy skin, hair, vision, and bones.

Including a few best foods like sweet potatoes, kale, and broccoli in your diet is a more efficient way to improve your diet immediately than eating vegetables with much less nutrient content.

The reason why you should eat vegetables daily is that vegetables provide dietary fiber, vitamins, minerals, and phytonutrients (*phyto* is a Greek word meaning "plant") like beta-carotene and lycopene, which are vital nutrients for maintaining the health of your body, preventing diseases, keeping your body younger, and allowing you to live longer. *USDA recommends a daily allowance of 2-3 cups of food from the vegetable food group for adults.*

The following is a list of some of the best vegetables commonly available in most groceries or supermarkets; they contain outstanding amounts of antioxidants, essential nutrients like fiber, and vitamins and minerals that keep the body healthy and prevent and reduce the risk of diseases. *The food nutrient data listed in this book are based on USDA National Nutrient Database for Standard Reference (Release 25). Percent Daily Values (%) recommended for nutrients is from FDA Daily Reference Values (2011) based on 2,000 calories intake per day, for adults or children four or more years of age.* [2,6]

Best Vegetables[2]

Sweet Potato	**Why Eat** Sweet potato lowers the risk of cancers and heart diseases, protects the eyes, and is strong anti-inflammatory. **Outstanding Facts** Eating only one hundred grams (3.5 ounces) will provide 384% daily needs for vitamin A (about eighteen times more than that of Broccoli), 33% for vitamin C, 25% for manganese, 14% for potassium, and 13% for dietary fiber. Vitamin A helps to reduce risk of heart disease, cancer, and helps to maintain healthy skin, hair, vision, and bones. Sweet potato is filled with carotenoid antioxidants, which prevent cancer and heart disease. The high amount of potassium helps to lower blood pressure. It is a good source of other vitamins like B6, pantothenic acid, and thiamin.
Kale	**Why Eat** It is one of the best vegetables, which has off-the-charts amounts of nutrients that prevent cancers; keep the eyes, heart, and bones healthy; and is strong anti-inflammatory. **Outstanding Facts** It contains plenty of antioxidants, which no vegetables can match. Foods with high antioxidants are the best to protect against heart diseases and cancers by

	cleaning up the free radicals that are associated with chronic human diseases. Free radicals are by-products that the body makes during metabolism. They cause diseases by triggering chain reactions that damage body cells. Eating only one hundred grams (3.5 ounces) will provide 272% of the daily requirement for vitamin A, 200% for vitamin C, a whopping 881% for vitamin K, and 33% for manganese. Vitamin A helps to reduce risk of heart disease, cancer, and helps to maintain healthy skin, hair, vision, and bones. Vitamin C is one of the most important vitamins; it fights infection, boosts the body's immune system, is critical for the healthy growth of body tissues, and protects the skin. Vitamin K is important for cardiovascular health and bone building. Kale is very rich in plant-based omega-3s and is a good source of other nutrients like calcium, magnesium, copper, potassium, and vitamin B6.
Broccoli	**Why Eat** Broccoli and other cruciferous vegetables like cauliflower and brussels sprouts are considered great must-have foods, which protect against many cancers, are anti-aging, and boost immune system. Eating once a week could lower the risk of cancer by 25% according to research. Eating cruciferous vegetables several times a week is recommended.

	Outstanding Facts Eating only one hundred grams (3.5 ounces) will provide 149% of the daily requirement for vitamin C, 127% for vitamin K, 16% for folate, and 12% for vitamin A. Vitamin C is one of the most important vitamins; it fights infection, boosts the body's immune system, is critical for healthy growth of body tissues, and protects the skin and teeth. Vitamin K is important for cardiovascular health and bone building. Broccoli has a very high amount of antioxidants. It contains the phytochemicals sulforaphane and indoles, which researchers identified to protect against cancers. Broccoli is a good source of other nutrients like manganese, dietary fiber, potassium, magnesium, calcium, vitamin B6, and iron.
Seaweed	**Why Eat** It is a nutrient-dense food from the sea; eating even a small amount could replenish nutrients that our bodies need to keep us healthy. **Outstanding Facts** Eating only one hundred grams (3.5 ounces) will provide 70% of the daily need for manganese, 49% for folate, 27% for magnesium, 15% for calcium, 14% for copper, and 12% for iron. Manganese is an essential mineral for bone health. It builds blood and other connective tissues, helps wound healing, and protects the body from the harm

	of free radicals. Folate is a B vitamin that plays a vital role for red blood cells development; reduces risk of heart disease, cancers, depression, and osteoporosis; protects pregnant women against birth defects; and improves brain function.
Spinach	**Why Eat** It is a superstar vegetable, which is good for the body in so many ways. Diet with plenty of spinach helps to prevent heart diseases and cancers, improves the immune system and brain functions, and is good for the skin and bones. **Outstanding Facts** It is one of the best sources for folate. Eating only one hundred grams (3.5 ounces) will provide 49% of the daily requirement for folate, 188% for vitamin A, 604% for vitamin K, 45% for manganese, 20% for magnesium, 16% for potassium, and 15% for iron. Vitamin A helps to reduce risk of heart disease and cancer and helps to maintain healthy skin, hair, vision, and bones. Vitamin K is important for cardiovascular health and bone building. Folate is a B vitamin that plays a vital role for red blood cells development; reduces risk of heart diseases, cancers, depression, and osteoporosis; protects pregnant women against birth defects; and improves brain function. Manganese is an essential mineral for bone health, builds blood and other connective tissues, helps wound healing, and protects the body from the harm of free radicals.

	Spinach contains plenty of antioxidants, which few vegetables can match. Foods with high antioxidants are the best to protect against heart diseases and cancers by cleaning up the free radicals that are associated with chronic human diseases.
Carrot	**Why Eat** It has plenty of vitamin A and carotenoids, which few vegetables can match. It is a great food, which prevents cancer and heart disease, is good for the eyesight, and is anti-inflammatory. **Outstanding Facts** It has plenty of vitamin A and Carotenoids, which few vegetables can match. Eating only one hundred grams (3.5 ounces) will provide 334% of the daily recommendation for vitamin A and an incredible amount of beta-carotene. Vitamin A helps to reduce risk of heart disease and cancer and helps to maintain healthy skin, hair, vision, and bones. Vitamin K is important for cardiovascular health and bone building. Beta-carotene converts to vitamin A during digestion and is one of the most powerful natural antioxidants, which helps to prevent cancers and promotes growth and development of the body. It is a good source of potassium, vitamins B, C, K, and dietary fiber. **How to Eat** Cooking carrots with oil will enhance the absorption of beta-carotene as carotene is fat soluble.

Red Bell Pepper	**Why Eat** It is a great food, which helps to decrease the risk of heart disease, cancer, arthritis, and eye disease and prevents cold. **Outstanding Facts** It is rich with antioxidants like vitamin C, beta-carotene, and lycopene. Eating only one hundred grams (3.5 ounces) will provide 213% of the daily recommendation for vitamin C, 63% for vitamin A, 12% for vitamin B6, and 11% for folate. Vitamin C is one of the most important vitamins; it fights infection, boosts the body's immune system, is critical for healthy growth of body tissues, and protects the skin. Vitamin A helps to reduce risk of heart disease and cancer and helps to maintain healthy skin, hair, vision, and bones. It has an incredible amount of beta-carotene, which is one of the most powerful natural antioxidants and helps to prevent cancers and promote growth and development of the body.
Cabbage	**Why Eat** It is a great food due to its richness in nutrients that prevent cancer, boost the immune system, and help in the body's detoxification. **Outstanding Facts** It is rich with vitamin K and C. Eating only one hundred grams (3.5 ounces) will provide nearly 95% of the daily requirement for vitamin K, 61% of your vitamin C, and 11% for folate. One hundred grams of

	cabbage contain only 25 calories. It is one of the ideal food choices for weight control. The glucosinolate found in cabbage has been shown to reduce the risk of cancer significantly by blocking the growth of certain types of cancers. Vitamin K is important for cardiovascular health and bone building. Vitamin C is one of the most important vitamins; it fights infection, boosts the body's immune system, is critical for healthy growth of body tissues, and protects the skin. It is a good source of plant-based omega-3s, calcium, potassium, iron, manganese, and dietary fiber.
Brussel Sprouts	**Why Eat** Brussel sprout is a top cruciferous vegetable originally from Brussels, Belgium. It has a very high antioxidant content, which protects against many cancers, is anti-aging, and boosts immunity. **Outstanding Facts** Eating only one hundred grams (3.5 ounces) will provide 103% of the daily requirement for vitamin C, 175% for vitamin K, 15% for folate, and 16% for vitamin A. Vitamin C is one of the most important vitamins; it fights infection, boosts the body's immune system, is critical for healthy growth of body tissues, and protects the skin and teeth. Vitamin K is important for cardiovascular health and bone building.

	Brussel sprouts contain plenty of antioxidants, which few vegetables can match. Foods with high antioxidants are the best to protect against heart diseases and cancers by cleaning up the free radicals that are associated with chronic human diseases. It is a good source of manganese, potassium, vitamins B6, dietary fiber, and iron.
Swiss Chard	**Why Eat** It is a great food packed with nutrients that prevent cancer, boost the immune system, and help in the body's detoxification. **Outstanding Facts** Eating only one hundred grams (3.5 ounces) will provide nearly 122% of the daily requirement for vitamin A, a whopping 1,038% for vitamin K, 50% of your vitamin C, 20% for magnesium, and 18% for manganese. Vitamin K is important for cardiovascular health and bone building. Vitamin A helps to reduce risk of heart disease and cancer and helps to maintain healthy skin, hair, vision, and bones. Vitamin C is one of the most important vitamins; it fights infection, boosts the body's immune system, is critical for healthy growth of body tissues, and protects the skin. It contains an incredible amount of lutein and zeaxanthin, which are carotenoids that protect the eyes.

Other healthy vegetables. Other than the best vegetables listed in the above table, there are many excellent vegetables that should be included in weekly vegetable choices:

Tomato	Tomato is a good source of lycopene, which is a carotenoid that is protective against cancers, heart diseases, and erectile dysfunction. Cooking tomato with oil will help enhance the body's absorption of lycopene.
	Tomato is a very good source of vitamin A, vitamin C, and vitamin K and a good source of potassium, manganese, folate, and vitamin B6.
Shiitake Mushroom	Shiitake mushrooms have shown in studies to have an antitumor effect, protecting against cardiovascular diseases and supporting the immune system.
	It is an excellent source of B vitamins riboflavin, niacin, and B6. It is rich in minerals like copper, potassium, magnesium, phosphorus, selenium, manganese, and zinc.
Cauliflower	Studies have shown that the antioxidant nutrients in cauliflower boost the body's detoxification, provide an anti-inflammatory effect, and protect against certain cancers.
	It is an excellent source of vitamin C and vitamin K. It is a very good source of folate, vitamin B6, dietary fiber, potassium, and manganese.

2.2 Best Fruit Choices

While most vegetables are edible parts of plants, fruits are the ovaries of plants. There are some fruits that are treated as vegetables traditionally, like various peppers, green beans, pumpkins, tomatoes, and cucumbers.

Like vegetables, fruits provide similar vital nutrients like dietary fiber, vitamins, minerals, and phytonutrients to our health. The basic differences between the nutritional values of fruits and vegetables are that vegetables generally have higher levels of vitamins and have important minerals like potassium, calcium, iron, while fruits tend to have higher levels of antioxidants. *The USDA recommended daily allowance is 1.5-2 cups of food from the fruit food group for adults.*

The following is a list of the best fruits commonly available, which have shown outstanding amounts of antioxidants (including beta-carotene), dietary fiber, vitamins, and other essential nutrients that keep the body healthy and prevent various diseases.

Best Fruits[2]

Blueberries	**Why Eat** Blueberries and other berries like blackberries, cranberries, raspberries, and strawberries are great must-eat fruits that have exceptionally high antioxidant content and anti-inflammatory compound, which provide protection against cancer, heart disease, stroke, and many other diseases. **Outstanding Facts** Blueberries have an impressive amount of health beneficial phytonutrients, which include anthocyanins antioxidant compounds that protect the plant against UV and are responsible for the bright colors of plants. Foods with high antioxidants are the best to protect against heart diseases and cancers by cleaning up the free radicals that are associated with chronic human diseases. Free radicals are by-products that the body makes during metabolism. They cause diseases by triggering chain reactions that damage body cells. Well-documented studies show that blueberries are anti-aging and anti-inflammatory and help to improve vision, memory, and brain function like cognitive problems associated with aging. Studies also show that eating blueberries helps to raise good HDL cholesterol and lower triglyceride. Other than antioxidants, eating only one hundred grams (3.5 ounces) will provide nearly 16% of the daily requirement for vitamin C, 24% for vitamin K, 17% for manganese, and 10% for dietary fiber.

Kiwi	**Why Eat** Kiwi is a superstar among fruits, with an outstanding amount of vitamin C content and an antioxidant capacity that protects from free-radical damage to human DNA. **Outstanding Facts** Studies show that eating kiwi daily is very heart healthy and helps to lower clot risk. The high level of the antioxidant lutein in kiwi is associated with eye health by lowering the risk of developing macular degeneration, which is a leading cause of impaired visions when people age. Orange juice has been recommended by doctors as a good source of vitamin C. Kiwi has almost twice the amount of vitamin C compared with orange. Eating only one hundred grams (3.5 ounces) will provide nearly 155% of the daily requirement for vitamin C, 50% of your vitamin K, and 12% for dietary fiber. Vitamin C is one of the most important vitamins; it fights infection, boosts the body's immune system, is critical for healthy growth of body tissues, and protects the skin. Kiwi is also a good source of potassium, vitamin E, enzymes, folate, magnesium, and copper.

Guava	**Why Eat** It is a truly great fruit by many standards. It has exceptionally high concentration of the antioxidant lycopene (higher than tomato), which provides protection against cancers, and other antioxidants that are essential for optimum health. **Outstanding Facts** It has amazingly more than four times the amount of vitamin C compared with orange. Eating one hundred grams (3.5 ounces) will provide nearly 381% of the daily requirement for vitamin C, 22% for dietary fiber, 12% for vitamin A, 12% for folate, and 12% for potassium. Vitamin C is one of the most important vitamins; it fights infection, boosts the body's immune system, is critical for healthy growth of body tissues, and protects the skin. The fiber content helps the prevention of diabetes and protection of the colon by decreasing exposure to toxins and harmful chemicals.
Apple	**Why Eat** Other than berries, apple is the fruit that ranks at the top with its antioxidant content. **Outstanding Facts** The abundance of polyphenols in apples provides a special benefit to the cardiovascular system by reducing platelet in the arteries and lowering risk of many chronic heart problems. Other health benefits of

	apples include being anti-asthma, reduction of lung cancer risk, and weight control due to its low glycemic index (GI) profile. Low GI foods are digested slowly and are associated with a gradual rise in blood-sugar levels.

Apple is a good source of vitamin C and dietary fiber, including the soluble fiber pectin. |
| Avocado | **Why Eat**
Avocado is a great fruit, which has off-the-charts amount of nutrients that lower cholesterol, prevent cancers, and are important for optimal health.

Outstanding Facts
It has the highest amount of heart-healthy monounsaturated fat among fruits. Monounsaturated fats in olive oil and avocado provide protection against heart disease by lowering bad LDL cholesterol and raising good HDL cholesterol.

Avocado has the highest amount of folate among fruits and has an incredible amount of dietary fiber. Eating one hundred grams (3.5 ounces) will provide nearly 27% of the daily requirement for dietary fiber, 17% for vitamin C, 35% for vitamin K, 20% for folate, 13% for vitamin B6, 14% for pantothenic acid, 14% for potassium, and 4% for protein (highest protein content than any other fruit).

The fiber content helps prevention of diabetes and protection of colon health by decreasing exposure to toxins and harmful chemicals in the colon. |

	Folate is a B vitamin that plays a vital role for red blood cells development; reduces risk of heart disease, cancers, depression, and osteoporosis; protects pregnant women against birth defects; and improves brain function. Studies have shown that eating vegetables with added avocados can help to absorb more nutrients than eating vegetables alone.
Papaya	**Why Eat** Papaya ranks highest among common fruits in terms of the overall amount of vitamins. The vitamins, enzymes, and other antioxidant nutrients in papaya help to maintain a healthy immune system and reduce inflammation. **Outstanding Facts** Eating one hundred grams (3.5 ounces) will provide 102% of the daily requirement for vitamin C, 19% for vitamin A, and 9% for folate. Vitamin C is one of the most important vitamins; it fights infection, boosts the body's immune system, is critical for healthy growth of body tissues, and protects the skin. Papaya is also a good source of potassium, dietary fiber, vitamin E, and the enzyme papain, which helps digestion.

Other healthy fruits. Other than the best fruits listed in the above table, there are many other excellent fruits that should be included in daily fruit choices.

Grapes	Grapes contain an abundance of antioxidants that are important for longevity. Studies show that flavonoids in grapes help to prevent heart disease and cancer and improve brain function. Grapes are a good source of vitamin C and K.
Watermelon	Watermelon is a top source of lycopene, which is a carotenoid that is protective against cancers, heart diseases, and erectile dysfunction. Watermelon is a good source of vitamin C and A.
Banana	Banana is a very good source of many nutrients, including vitamin C, vitamin B6, potassium, manganese, and dietary fiber, which are important for optimal health. Potassium in banana helps to lower high blood pressure.
Orange and Other Citrus Fruits	Citrus fruits contain many phytochemicals that have been shown to have an anti-inflammatory effect and help reduce the risk of cancers. Orange is an excellent source of vitamin C and a good source of dietary fiber, folate, thiamin, vitamin A, and calcium.

2.3 Best Grains

Eating whole grains is an important part of a healthy diet. Grains are fruits of the grass family and the most important food plants for humans. The best and healthiest kinds of grains are whole grains. There are many scientific researches that show eating whole grains reduces risk of diabetes and cardiovascular diseases by over 20%.[3,4] Cardiovascular conditions, including heart disease and stroke, account for one-third of deaths worldwide.

Choosing whole grains over refined grain is one of the smartest things that people could do to improve their diets. Well-known whole grains like oatmeal that are full of soluble fiber help to lower bad LDL cholesterol.

The reason to eat refined grains less is that refined grains like white bread, white rice, and white flour have lost all the fiber and most of the nutrients like vitamin E and B (folate, thiamin, riboflavin, niacin) and minerals (iron, magnesium) during the refining process. Other than losing the most nutritious parts, refined grains are mostly starches, which are easily converted to blood sugar and send blood-sugar levels soaring.

Whole grains retain the entire grain seed, which include the bran, germ, and the endosperm, while refined grains are mostly endosperm. Endosperm is energy dense and a good source of energy for our daily activities. But it is the nutrient-poor portion of the grain. Most of the nutrients of grains like fiber, vitamins, antioxidants, phytonutrients, and vitamins and minerals reside in the bran and germ components.

The difference would be very significant when you choose to eat whole grains or refined grains on a daily basis. Completely switching from refined grains to whole grains is definitely a key step toward a healthy diet and can be very straightforward: starting with whole-grain oatmeal or cereal for breakfast, eating whole-grain bread or whole wheat pasta instead of white bread or white-flour pasta, or eating brown or wild rice instead of white rice.

All whole grains are very healthy and provide similar nutrients, like fiber, vitamins, and minerals. Commonly available whole grain foods include brown rice, wild rice, oatmeal, whole wheat flour, barley, quinoa, amaranth, bulgur, couscous, and kasha. *The USDA recommended daily allowance is 3-4 ounces of food from the grain food group for adults.*

The following is a list of the best whole grains, which contain exceptionally high contents of phytonutrients that are essential to health and help to protect the body and fight diseases.

Best Grains

Oats	**Why Eat** Oats are superstar whole grains, which have an exceptional amount of fiber, very high protein, and are rich in minerals. Oats are well known for lowering the bad cholesterol (LDL) due to the soluble fiber beta glucan. **Outstanding Facts** Eating only one hundred grams (3.5 ounces) will provide 42% of the daily recommendation for dietary fiber, will provide 26% for iron and zinc, 31% for copper, 44% for magnesium, and an amazing 246% of the daily recommendation for manganese. Manganese is an essential mineral for bone health. It builds blood and other connective tissues, helps wound healing, and protects the body from the harm of free radicals. Fiber is important for the health of the digestive system and for lowering cholesterol. It is also good for binding and removing toxins from the colon and helps the body regulate blood sugar. Oats are also a great source of B vitamins like thiamin, folate, riboflavin, and pantothenic acid. Oats take a long time to digest and leave you feeling satisfied for a longer time. They are an ideal food for anyone trying to lose weight.

Quinoa	**Why Eat** Pronounced *keen-wa*. This grain, rooted in South America, is a true supergrain, providing complete protein, which most other grains lack, and it is striking with its overall nutrient richness. **Outstanding Facts** Quinoa protein is considered a complete protein source, like meats or eggs, which has the adequate proportion of all nine of the essential amino acids. It contains all kinds of minerals like manganese, potassium, phosphorus, copper, iron, and magnesium which makes it an effective agent against cancer and heart disease, and it is anti-inflammatory. It is also great source of vitamin B like folate, thiamin, riboflavin, B6 and vitamin E. It has an exceptionally low glycemic index, which means that they release sugar into the blood very slowly and could play a key role in the active prevention of diabetes.
Amaranth	**Why Eat** Originating from Africa, it is one of the smallest grains in the world, but it is a supergrain, which has an exceptionally high amount of protein and is very rich with all kinds of highly nutritious minerals, like manganese, iron, potassium, phosphorus, magnesium, and selenium. **Outstanding Facts** Amaranth protein is considered a complete protein source, like meat or eggs, which has the adequate proportion of all nine of the essential amino acids.

	It is gluten free and has an exceptionally low glycemic index (GI), which means that they release sugar into the blood very slowly and could play a key role in the active prevention of diabetes.
Teff	**Why Eat** Originating from Northeast Africa, it is the smallest grain and one of the tastier grains in the world. It is a true superstar whole grain, which has an exceptional amount of protein, fiber, and the highest amount of highly nutritious minerals among all grains. **Outstanding Facts** Eating only one hundred grams (3.5 ounces) will provide 32% of the daily recommendation for dietary fiber; an amazing 462% of the daily recommendation for manganese, which is an essential mineral for bone health and builds blood and other connective tissues; over 40% for iron, magnesium, copper, and phosphorus. Manganese is an essential mineral for bone health. It builds blood and other connective tissues, helps wound healing, and protects the body from the harm of free radicals. It contains a high level of amino acid composition, which helps to maintain a strong body immune system.
Kamut	**Why Eat** Pronounced *ka-moot*. It is a supergrain and is actually wheat. It has exceptionally high protein and is packed with all kinds of minerals, like manganese, iron, potassium, phosphorus, magnesium, and selenium.

> **Outstanding Facts**
>
> Eating only one hundred grams (3.5 ounces) will provide 25% of the daily recommendation for iron and zinc, 26% for copper, 34% for magnesium, 99% for selenium, and an amazing 143% of the daily recommendation for manganese.
>
> It is also great source of B vitamins, like thiamin (39% of the daily recommendation), niacin (32% of the daily recommendation), vitamin B6, riboflavin, and pantothenic acid.

2.4 Best Protein Foods

Other than water, protein is the most plentiful substance in our bodies. Every body cell, muscle, skin, hair, enzymes, bones, and various body organs have a substantial amount of protein. To build, maintain, and replace the proteins in our bodies, we need to eat protein foods, which are digested into amino acids, used to create protein. Eating sufficient protein foods is vital for the health and maintenance of our bodies.

To make all types of proteins that the body needs, our bodies require twenty different amino acids, and nine of them are called essential amino acids. They are considered essential because that they must come from food and cannot be made by our bodies.

Animals and plants are the two main sources for the protein food group. Foods from animal sources like meat, poultry, seafood, and eggs are considered complete protein sources because they include all nine essential amino acids, which our bodies need.

Foods from plant sources like grains (rice, wheat, oat, and corn), legumes (beans, peas, lentils, and soybeans), seeds, and nuts (walnuts and almonds) are mostly considered as incomplete protein sources because they are missing one or more of the nine essential amino acids. Quinoa and amaranth in the best grains list are the few exceptions and are complete protein foods. But eating two of any plant groups (grains, legumes, seeds, and nuts) will make a complete protein diet because the combination will provide adequate amounts of all the essential amino acids.

What makes a food a good protein food is the nutrients other than protein that the food contains. The protein food group provides more than just the protein. Foods in the protein food group provide vital nutrients that are important for the health of the body. Beans are considered the best plant-based protein foods, with the highest fiber and antioxidants content. Seafood, like salmons, is the best source of omega-3, which is good for the heart and rich in phosphorus, iron, potassium, vitamin B6, and niacin.

The USDA recommended daily allowance is 5-6.5 ounce of food from the protein food group for adults (higher daily allowance than other food groups). The following is the list of best foods among the protein group.

Best Proteins

Small Red Bean	**Why Eat** Small red bean is a great food, which is rich with antioxidant and healthy dietary fiber, providing protection against cancer, heart disease, stroke, and many other diseases. **Outstanding Facts** Small red bean is at the top of the list of common plant foods regarding antioxidant content. Foods with high antioxidants are anti-aging and are the best to protect against heart diseases and cancers by cleaning up the free radicals that are associated with chronic human diseases. Free radicals are by-products that the body makes during metabolism. They cause diseases by triggering chain reactions that damage body cells. Small red bean is a fiber all-star, rich in dietary fiber. Eating only one hundred grams (3.5 ounces) will provide an impressive 30% of the daily recommendation for dietary fiber and 16% for iron. Dietary fiber is important for the health of the digestive system and for lowering cholesterol. It is also good for binding and removing toxins from the colon and helps blood sugar regulation in diabetes. It is a rich source of various minerals, like magnesium, phosphorus, potassium, copper, manganese, and calcium. Red bean is also a good source of various vitamins, like folate, thiamin, and vitamin B6.

	Other beans like red kidney bean and pinto bean have a very similar health benefits profile like the small red bean.
Walnut	**Why Eat** It is one of the best sources of plant protein and one of the most nutrient-dense foods, with impressive health benefits. **Outstanding Facts** The nutrient content of walnut is so impressive that few other foods can match it. Eating a small handful of walnut a day can replenishes nutrients that our bodies need to keep us healthy. It has an incredible amount of omega-3 content, which is protective to the heart and circulation. Nearly 90% of walnut fats are valuable, heart-healthy monounsaturated and polyunsaturated fats (the same type of fats as in olive oil). Eating one hundred grams (3.5 ounces) will provide 15.2 grams of protein (versus 22 grams for salmon), nearly 27% of the daily requirement for fiber, an amazing 171% of the daily recommendation for manganese, 79% for copper, 40% for magnesium, 35% for phosphorus, 21% for zinc, 16% for iron, and 10% for calcium. It is an excellent source of vitamins, like folate (25%), thiamin (23%), and vitamin B6 (27%). Studies have shown that eating a handful of walnuts regularly will greatly reduce risk of heart disease, diabetes, cancer, and other chronic ailments; improve memory and other brain functions; and even improve sperm quality for men.

Almond	**Why Eat** It is a nutrient-dense top food, which is packed with plant protein, dietary fiber, monounsaturated fat, and other great nutrients. **Outstanding Facts** Nearly 92% of almond fats are valuable, heart-healthy monounsaturated and polyunsaturated fats (the same type of fats as in olive oil). Eating one hundred grams (3.5 ounces) will provide 21.2 grams of protein (versus 22 grams for salmon), 49% of the daily requirement for dietary fiber, 114% for manganese, 50% for copper, 67% for magnesium, 48% for phosphorus, 26% for calcium, 21% for zinc, and 21% for iron. It is also an excellent source of the antioxidant vitamin E (87% of the daily requirement) and other vitamins like riboflavin (60%), niacin (17%), thiamin (14%), and folate (12%). Studies have shown that eating a handful of almonds regularly will lower LDL and reduce risk of cardiovascular disease and diabetes.
Quinoa	**Why Eat** It is a supergrain, containing more protein than any other grain. Quinoa protein is considered as complete protein and is gluten free. It is also packed with many nutrients. See best grain list for details.

Salmon	**Why Eat** Salmon is the perfect protein superfood, containing an outstanding amount of omega-3, healthy fats, and essential minerals and vitamins, which protect against heart disease, inflammation, depression, and joint pain. **Outstanding Facts** Salmon contains an incredible amount of omega-3 fatty acids, which are anti-inflammatory, reduce the risk of blood clots, improve cholesterol level, and help to prevent heart attacks. Eating one hundred grams (3.5 ounces) will provide 22 grams of protein (44% of the daily requirement), provide nearly 59% for selenium, 25% for phosphorus, 47% for vitamin B12, 40% for niacin, 32% for vitamin B6, and 23% for thiamin. The high amount of selenium in salmon is particularly important for reducing risk of joint inflammation and cardiovascular disease and aids in the prevention of cancers. Its richness in minerals is also important for healthier skin, hair, and nails.
Anchovy	**Why Eat** Anchovy is a nutrient-dense food, which is packed with protein, a good source of omega-3 (same as salmon), heart-healthy fats, and essential minerals and vitamins, helping to protect against heart disease, inflammation, depression, and joint pain.

> **Outstanding Facts**
>
> Anchovy contains an incredible amount of omega-3 fatty acids, which are anti-inflammatory, reduce the risk of blood clots, improve cholesterol level, and help to prevent heart attacks.
>
> Eating one hundred grams (3.5 ounces) will provide 28.9 grams of protein (58% of the daily requirement), provide 97% of the daily requirement for selenium, 100% for niacin, 26% for iron, 25% for phosphorus, 23% for calcium, 21% for riboflavin, and 11% for vitamin E.

2.5 Best Foods in Other Food Groups

There are some well-known best foods that provide unique health benefits but do not belong to any of the four food groups (vegetables, fruits, grains, and proteins).

Healthy oils are such an example. Oils are considered as an important part of diet because healthy oils are highly anti-inflammatory, are major sources of vitamin E and vitamin K, have plenty of plant phenols with potent antioxidant properties, provide good polyunsaturated or monounsaturated fats (which contain essential fatty acids that reduce bad LDL cholesterol), and are good for the heart. *The USDA recommended daily allowance is 5-7 teaspoons of oils for adults.*

Other than healthy oils, dark chocolates, yogurt, maple syrup, and red wine are among the best foods that belong to the other food groups.

Best Foods in the Other Food Group

Olive Oil	**Why Eat** Olive oil is a great natural food, containing components that provide many health and anti disease benefits. **Outstanding Facts** Seventy-six percent of fat in olive oil are monounsaturated fatty acids. Studies have shown that the very high content of monounsaturated fats in olive oil provide protection against heart disease by lowering bad LDL cholesterol and raising good HDL cholesterol. The plant phenols with potent antioxidant properties in olive oil improve blood circulation and protect blood vessels and cardiac tissues. FDA permits foods containing olive oil to carry the label "May reduce the risk of coronary heart disease." Coronary heart disease is the leading cause of death in the United States, which is caused by the buildup of plaque and hardening of the arteries to the heart. The plant phenols provide protection against high blood pressure, diabetes, and cancers. The antioxidants and anti-inflammatory effects of olive oil also provide prevention or reduction of the severity of arthritis and asthma. Virgin olive oil, which is not further refined, has a higher level of phenols than more refined olive oil. Extra-virgin olive oil (EVOO) that is cold-pressed is the best. Most mass-produced olive oils are extracted with chemical solvents, but the best natural extraction method is cold-pressing.

	When cooking, the smoking point of olive oil varieties should be considered. EVVO has the lowest smoking point, which is 406°F (Bertolli® brand). Olive oil has a smoking point of 460°F (Bertolli® brand). Virgin olive oil has a smoking point between these two oils. Toxic fumes and harmful radicals will be produced when oils are heating above their smoke points. The smoking points of most olive oils are above the recommended temperature of 350°F-370°F for frying foods.
Yogurt	**Why Eat** Organic, plain yogurt contains a high level of protein, with balanced amounts of carbohydrates and essential vitamins and minerals. **Outstanding Facts** It has a high content of bone-healthy calcium. One cup of yogurt will provide 40-50% of most people's daily needs for calcium. What makes yogurt a superfood is that it is one of the best probiotic foods, containing healthy active bacteria, with the power to protect the body in myriad ways. The bacteria in yogurt help to inhibit the growth of harmful bacteria and increase the absorption of calcium and B vitamins, boost the immune system, enhance digestion, and fight infection.
Dark Chocolate	**Why Eat** Chocolate is a favorite food for many people and is also good for the heart's health. Studies have shown that eating a moderate amount of chocolates, especially dark chocolates, helps cardiovascular health and lowers the risk of stroke.

	Outstanding Facts Plenty of flavonoids found in chocolates are found to be especially helpful in protecting the blood vessel and preventing high blood pressure through the antioxidant and anti-inflammatory properties of these said flavonoids. Foods with high antioxidants are anti-aging and the best to protect against heart disease and cancers by cleaning up the free radicals that are associated with chronic human diseases. Free radicals are by-products that the body makes during metabolism. They cause diseases by triggering chain reactions that damage body cells.
Maple Syrup	**Why Eat** Organic maple syrup is a natural sweetener packed with anti-inflammatory and antioxidant content. **Outstanding Facts** Studies have found 54 amazing beneficial phenolic compounds[5] in maple syrup, including five that are only unique in maple syrup. The others are the same as found in berries, green tea, flax seeds, and red wines. The phenolic compounds help fight cancer, diabetes, and are anti-inflammatory. Inflammations are associated with most chronic diseases. One ounce (28 grams) of maple syrup provides 46% of the daily requirement for manganese and 8% for zinc. Manganese is an essential mineral for bone health. It builds blood and other connective tissues, boosts the immune system, helps wound healing, and protects the body from the harm of free radicals. Zinc is a mineral that promotes men's prostate health.

Red Wine	**Why Eat** Drinking red wine is a great enjoyment for many people and is also good for the heart's health. Studies have shown that drinking a moderate amount of red wine weekly is particularly heart protective. **Outstanding Facts** Unique phytonutrients, particularly resveratrol, found in red wine have been widely studied and found to be especially helpful in protecting the blood vessels, reducing risk of inflammation and blood clotting, lowering bad LDL, and increasing good HDL through the antioxidant and anti-inflammatory properties of the said phytonutrients. Foods with high antioxidants are anti-aging and are the best to protect against heart diseases and cancers by cleaning up the free radicals that are associated with chronic human diseases. Free radicals are by-products that the body makes during metabolism. They cause diseases by triggering chain reactions that damage body cells.

2.6 Summary

1. Wellbeing is not just about weight loss; it is about the absence of disease, being free of pains, having youthfulness, longevity, and your body being in a state filled with energy and vitality, where you are able to enjoy food and life to the fullest extent. Eating the best foods is the most direct and efficient way to improve your diet immediately. When you eat the healthiest foods that give your body the most nutrient benefits, you also leave less room for unhealthy foods. Eating the Best Food is a strategy to help you achieve advanced level of diet in the most efficient way.

2. David Murdock is a great example that shows we could eat wisely to have an energetic and vibrant life, free of major diseases or minor ailments. Murdock did not start his healthy diet until his sixties. It is never too late to start for anyone. The best foods are mostly unprocessed, real foods and are available in your local supermarkets. The proactive diet approach (PDA) provides a list of best choices for each major food group (also available in Appendix A).

    - Best Vegetable Choices
    - Best Fruit Choices
    - Best Grains
    - Best Protein Foods
    - Best Foods in Other Foods Group

3. Pick one food to start your journey to wellbeing. Very few individuals have the willpower to just switch to healthy foods and abandon all the bad foods in one day and stick with the new diet. But it is realistic for most people to add just one of the best foods that they truly enjoy. Most of the best foods are tasty and enjoyable. Start slowly, adding one food to your

weekly diet, and stick with the change, then move on to the next food once you become comfortable. With each new best food added to your weekly diet, you would also have less room for bad food. This small and incremental approach does not cause the stress or guilt that is commonly associated with other diet programs. Because you are always making progress, and you get immediate reward physically and mentally with every small improvement. Over time, the approach will truly accomplish what many other diet recommendations had failed to do, a lifelong healthy diet habit.

CHAPTER 3

Avoid the Worst Foods

In year 2011, there was an amazing story in tennis. Novak Djokovic ascended to become the world's most dominant tennis player and the world's best athlete of 2011 after four years as no. 3 player in the world. His opponents were two of the greatest and almost unbeatable players in tennis history. Rafael Nadal was in his prime at the young age of twenty-five, with ten grand titles already under his belt; and all-time great, seventeen times grand-slam winner thirty-year-old Roger Federer was still at his peak performance. The near-miraculous improvement in a short period that elevated Djokovic from no. 3 in the world to a convincing great player was because physically he became stronger and had more energy at court due to a simple change of diet. Several months before 2011, his nutritionist and doctor identified that he was allergic to gluten, a protein that is found among foods with flours, like pizza, pasta, and breads, which Djokovic had fed his body daily. Gluten is the cause of various medical issues. It is a protein found in grains, such as wheat, barley, and rye. Baked foods and grains are known to be rich with gluten.

The change to Djokovic's diet is quite simple. Djokovic totally avoided eating gluten foods as a caution. But the impact was very big. He slept much better. The result was nothing short of astounding on the tennis court. He became sharper at court and mentally confident, and what he had achieved in 2011 was the single best year for any tennis player in history.

Djokovic was a very good tennis player prior to his diet change. But the improvement of his diet and sleep had made him a great one. The story of Djokovic is that diet plays a critical role to the performance of a world-class athlete. Regardless who we are or what we believe, there is a consequence of what we eat. Eating healthy foods positively affects the quality of our daily life like how we feel, our daily energy level, and our brain function and improves our defense against chronic diseases. Eating unhealthy foods has the opposite effect from causing minor ailments to bringing major diseases.

Researches and scientific facts are very clear that unhealthy diets are the leading causes of human death. *When people get sick frequently or get major illnesses, the most important question they need to ask is what caused the illness.* Diet habits and other lifestyle factors are very likely to be the main cause of most ailments of the body. Cardiovascular diseases, including heart disease and stroke, are the number one cause of human death and cancers are the number two leading cause of death in Western countries. According to the World Health Organization, at least 30% of cancers are due to dietary factors. Unhealthy diets, physical inactivity, and smoking are responsible for about 80% of cardiovascular diseases.

People are aware more or less that the foods that they choose to eat are unhealthy when they are eating donuts, hamburgers, sugary soda, french fries, red meats, and processed foods like bacon and hot dogs. *But most people do not know that what they are eating are some of the worst foods.*

For people who like to live free of diseases, avoiding unhealthy foods is a must. The most effective and smart way to achieve this goal is for people to avoid those most harmful foods, which are clearly linked to major human diseases. Second, people should reduce or replace those foods that are likely to be eaten in large quantities and frequently but have minimal nutrient value, or even have negative health effects, so that they have more room for best foods.

There could be only two consequences of eating any food: net positive or net negative to our health. This book categorizes foods that should be avoided into two categories: most harmful foods and undesirable foods.

3.1 Most Harmful Foods

Most harmful foods are the most net negative foods. They are the kinds of foods that are linked directly to major human diseases like cancer, heart disease, and diabetes mostly because of harmful chemical compounds, high content of unhealthy fats, salts, and sugars in those foods.

In 2012, the World Cancer Research Fund (WCRF)[1] published a very comprehensive report on the evidence of the link of cancer to diet, body weight, and physical activity. The report found convincing evidence linking excess body fat and eating processed meat and red meat to higher cancer risk. Excess body fats are mostly caused by high intake of fats, calories, and sugars in diets.

High intake of saturated fats, trans fat, and high sugars and sodium is the major factor causing high blood pressure, raising bad cholesterol and blood glucose, and bringing about heart disease and diabetes. Sugar has a high caloric content. High sugar intake causes weight gain, is associated with insulin resistance, and encourages inflammation and infection. Heart disease is the number one cause of death for both men and women in America. Thirty-five percent of Americans today are considered obese,[2] and 25.8 million (8.35%) of Americans have diabetes.[3]

Avoiding these most harmful foods is the best action you can take to improve your diet, your weight, and your current and future health.

Most Harmful Foods

Processed Meats	**Why Avoid** There are strong evidences that eating processed meats increases risk of cancers, heart diseases, and diabetes. **Outstanding Facts** In 2012, after studying more than seven thousand clinical studies, the World Cancer Research Fund (WCRF)[1] advised people to avoid processed meats for a lifetime because of convincing evidences that processed meats increase the risk of colorectal cancer. Risk of colorectal cancer increases by 21% for every 1.7 ounces of processed meat intake. A study published in 2010 in the journal *Circulation* also concluded that eating processed foods raised the risk of heart disease and diabetes.[4] The risk of heart disease increases by 42% and the risk of diabetes increases by 19% for every two ounces of processed meat intake. Processed meats are mostly red meats that are preserved by the addition of preservatives, salt, or by smoking or curing. *They include bacon, sausage, ham, hot dogs, deli meat, pepperoni, and salami.* Even though the link between eating processed meats and cancers is very strong, there are controversies regarding whether the chemical sodium nitrite, commonly used in processed foods for preservative purposes, cause the cancers. The FDA and USDA have deemed them safe when within the law's specified limits.

Starchy Foods in High Temperature	**Why Avoid** Starchy foods in high temperature produce a chemical called acrylamide. Acrylamide has been shown to cause cancer in animal studies. A 2007 Dutch study[5] involving 62,000 women linked high acrylamide intake in diet to higher risk of womb and ovarian cancers. **Outstanding Facts** Swedish scientists in 2002 first discovered that the chemical acrylamide was formed when starchy foods were fried or baked at high temperatures above 248°F (120°C). Acrylamide was not found when starchy foods were prepared below this temperature or non-starchy foods in high temperatures. *Potato chips and french fries* are the top sources of acrylamide intake by the American population. Other top acrylamide foods include breakfast cereals, crackers, coffee, and toast. The Environmental Protection Agency (EPA)[6] set the acceptable limit of the amount of acrylamide level to 0.5ppb in drinking water due to the increased risk of getting cancer and the potential problem to the nerve system or the blood several decades ago. According to the Food and Drug Administration (FDA) data, some potato chips and nachos contain up to several thousand times the limit of EPA. Most french fries, some crackers, and most wheat cereals contain a several hundred times higher amount of acrylamide than the EPA limit.

	FDA has not advised consumers to avoid foods with acrylamide due to incomplete evidence linking dietary acrylamide intake to human cancer risk. However, Canada and the European Union placed acrylamide on their list of hazardous substances after their own studies.
Meats in High Temperature	**Why Avoid** Meats in high temperature produce the chemicals HCAs (heterocyclic amines) and PAHs (polycyclic aromatic hydrocarbons). HCAs and PAHs are included in the list of known carcinogens and found to increase cancer risks. **Outstanding Facts** HCAs are formed when meats are cooked at high temperatures (grilled or pan fried) above 300ºF or are cooked for a long time. Amino acids and the protein creatine in meats form HCAs when meats are under high temperatures. PAHs are formed when meats are under direct flame and exposed to smoke or charring. *Skinless chicken breast, steak, pork, salmon with skin, and hamburger* are the top five worst meats to grill, which contain very high levels of HCAs according to the Cancer Project[7] dietitians. Skinless chicken breast is the worst, with more than ten times HCAs than steak when grilled. The more done and longer the time the meats are under high temperatures, the higher amounts of HCAs would form.

Trans Fats	**Why Avoid**
	Trans fats are considered to be the worst fats, which are very harmful to the heart, raising bad LDL cholesterol, raising artery-clogging lipoprotein and triglyceride, and lowering good HDL cholesterol.
	Facts
	Trans fats are artificially produced through a hydrogenation process wherein hydrogen is added to natural vegetable oil under heated condition turn liquid oils into solid fat at room temperature to prolong the shelf life of the oil.
	Trans fats are inexpensive. Food manufacturers and restaurants use them to increase the shelf life of foods and enhance food texture and stability.
	Over 80% of trans fats exist in processed foods. According to the Centers for Disease Control (CDC) and the Federal Drug Administration (FDA),[8] *foods containing the most trans fats are microwave popcorn, cookies and crackers, bakeries, frozen pies and pizzas, breakfast cereals, margarines, and coffee creamers.*
	Foods with labels of "zero trans fats" do not mean they have no trans fats. *FDA allows foods to be labeled "zero grams trans fats" if they contain only up to 0.49 grams of trans fat per serving.*
	FDA requires all food manufacturers to include trans fats on nutrition labels. New York City and a dozen other states and cities have banned restaurants from serving foods containing more than 0.5 grams of trans fat per serving.

	Avoiding processed foods high in trans fats is a must for a healthy diet.

3.2 Undesirable Foods

Undesirable foods are foods that provide a net negative or a small net positive to health but are likely to be eaten in high quantity and frequently. When people eat more foods with little nutritional values, they will have less room for more healthier and disease-fighting foods.

Reducing or replacing these foods in the diet is a smart way to improve diet to reach a higher level.

Undesirable Foods List

Fast Foods	**Why Avoid** Many fast foods are very unhealthy in so many ways. Chemicals added to the foods, high amount of unhealthy fats and sodium, processed meats, and cooking methods are what make them very bad for the health. **Outstanding Facts** To keep prices low for consumers, typical fast-food meals are made with highly processed ingredients, and many are fried with cheap but very unhealthy oils. Other than feeding hunger and satisfying craving, most fast-food meals provide very little nutrients and are packed with high amounts of saturated and trans fat, sodium, and many unhealthy food additives.

	According to the Web site of one of the top hamburger restaurants in the United States, *a large serving of fries contains 71 grams of fats (16 grams are saturated fats) and a whopping 1,474 calories.* USDA recommends only 27-36 grams of fats daily for normal adults. A bacon cheeseburger from the same hamburger restaurant provides 920 calories and 62 grams of fats (29.5 grams are saturated fats). The fats are responsible for 560 of 920 calories. High calories lead to being overweight. High saturated fat intake has been linked to coronary heart disease and diabetes. Trans fats are the worst fat and considered very harmful to the heart, raising bad LDL cholesterol, raising artery-clogging lipoprotein and triglyceride, and lowering good HDL cholesterol. High sodium leads to high blood pressure and is a major cause of cardiovascular diseases.
Refined Grains	**Why Avoid** Refined grains miss the health benefits provided by whole grains and cause spike and crash of blood-sugar levels, which is not healthy to the heart and one's mood. **Outstanding Facts** Refined grains like white bread, regular white pasta, and white rice contain almost zero fiber and have lost most of their healthy nutrients like vitamins and minerals during the refining process; while *whole grains reduce risk of diabetes and cardiovascular diseases by over 20%.*

	Refined grains are mostly starches, which are easily converted to blood sugar and send blood sugar levels soaring and crashing.

Most white flour in the United States contains the carcinogenic ingredient potassium bromate, which is a flour improver that causes the flour to rise higher in the oven and strengthens the dough. It is used by food manufacturers to increase volume in white flour, reduce time for baking, and save cost.

While bromates are banned in EU, Canada, and many other countries, only California in the United States requires that potassium bromate be listed with a warning label. |
| Sugar | **Why Avoid**
The obesity rate among American adults is 35% today. There is a direct link between high sugar intake to being overweight, the rate of obesity, and type II diabetes.

Outstanding Facts
The average American eats over 142 pounds of added sugar per year according to USDA.[9] Sugar is found in almost all processed foods. Soft drinks, prepared and canned foods, and sweetened fruit drinks are the top sources of added sugar.

The massive intake of sugar is what makes sugar detrimental to the health. It is a major factor in obesity and diabetes. |

	Sugar is added to foods to make them tastier, and people end up eating much more. High calories are generated from high sugar consumption and are eventually converted to fat in the body. One 12 oz can of cola contains about ten teaspoons (40 grams) of sugar.
Red Meats	**Why Avoid** Red meat from conventionally raised animals contains high amounts of saturated fat and cholesterol. There are convincing evidences that eating red meat (beef, lamb, and pork) increases risk of cancers and heart diseases. **Outstanding Facts** In 2012, after studying more than 7,000 clinical studies, the World Cancer Research Fund (WCRF)[1] advised people to limit meats because of convincing evidence that red meats increase the risk of cancers. The American Institute for Cancer Research recommends limiting intake of red meat to no more than eighteen ounces per week.[10] Studies suggested the cancer risk rises when the amount of red meat consumed is beyond this amount. In 2012, a study published by *Archives of Internal Medicine*[11] found that red meat consumption was associated with an increased risk of cardiovascular death, cancer, and overall death.

Other than the foods in the above two lists, there are still many unhealthy foods that dieters should stay away from.

Canned Foods	Unhealthy ingredients include high sodium, high level of bisphenol A (BPA), and preservatives.
Chips, Crackers, Cookies	Unhealthy ingredients include hydrogenated and rancid oil, trans fats, acrylamide, and food additives.
Ice Cream	Unhealthy ingredients include sugar, fat, and additives for artificial color and taste.
Donuts	Unhealthy ingredients include sugar, vegetable shortening, white flour, acrylamide, and food additives.

3.3 Summary

1. Avoiding eating the most unhealthy and harmful foods which give us minor ailments or major illnesses like heart diseases, cancers, and diabetes is an essential and smart thing to do to live an active, satisfying, and vibrant life free of diseases. Instead of eating the harmful foods to give yourself diseases and looking for the best doctor and medicines later, a healthy diet incorporating the best foods in every group will have a positive impact to your mood, empower your body's defense against various diseases, and improve the overall wellbeing of your life.

2. Summary of foods to avoid

    The book provides a list of the most harmful foods and a list of the most undesirable foods that people should avoid (also available in Appendix B).

Most Harmful Foods: Absolutely no processed meats like hot dog, deli meat, ham, and bacons. Avoid fried starchy foods, avoid grilled or barbecued meats, be cautious about any fried foods, and avoid sweet or sugary soda.

Undesirables Foods: Limit red meats to no more than 18 ounces per week. Replace with deepwater fishes (like salmon and tuna) and other protein-rich foods (like red beans, lentils, and tofu).

Be extra cautious about fast foods; or better yet, totally avoid them. Avoid fried starchy foods like french fries and avoid fried meats like fried chickens. Go to fast-food places that offer foods with healthy ingredients.

Reduce or replace refined grains by whole grains. Instead of white rice, choose brown rice or the best grains like quinoa, oats, and amaranth. Replace white bread and white pasta with whole grain bread and pasta.

3. Pick one food to give up. It is very difficult or almost impossible for most people to abandon all the bad foods from their diet in one day. But it is realistic for most people to pick just one of the worst foods that they feel is easy to give up. Start slowly with one food to avoid and stick with the change, then move on to the next food after you get comfortable. This gradual approach sounds simple, but the result could be very significant. Over time, the approach will truly accomplish what many other diet recommendations had failed to do, keeping the bad foods from the diet permanently.

4. Do not get near bad foods. When you go to restaurants that carry unhealthy food options, it is very hard to avoid the bad foods. Always try to go to restaurants that offer healthy options. When shopping for groceries, try not to put unhealthy foods in

the shopping cart. When you do not have unhealthy foods at home, you and your family would eat less of them. Associate with people who eat healthy foods or live healthy lifestyles. Research found that people close to you have very big influence to your food choices.

5. Many people have the false assumption that they would be fine to eat unhealthy foods because they go to the gym regularly. The fact is that rigorous exercise daily or other activities can't compensate for the harm from routinely eating unhealthy foods.

CHAPTER 4

Achieve Life-Long Healthy Weight

4.1 Obesity Cancer Risk and Epidemic

In 2012, the World Cancer Research Fund (WCRF)[1] and the American Institute for Cancer Research (AICR) published the results of a very systematic assessment of the link of cancer to food nutrition, physical activity, and body weight. The *most authoritative* ever report on cancer risk is based on five years of review and assessment by the top researchers in the world of over more than seven thousand clinical studies regarding evidence of the link of cancer to various diets, physical activities, sedentary living, and being breast-fed.

The number one recommendation from this landmark WCRF report is to avoid excessive body fatness. Among all the factors evaluated for evidence of link to cancer, ***body fatness is found convincingly linked to six cancers*** (*pancreas, kidney, postmenopausal breast, colorectum, esophagus, and endometrium*) more than any other factors. It is also found as a probable cause of gallbladder cancer. The evidence linking body fatness to many cancers is deemed convincing in this report, not just probable cause or unclear or inconclusive.

For many years, studies have established link of obesity to higher risk of heart diseases and diabetes. The fact is clear that very few obese individuals have healthy normal cholesterol, normal blood sugar, or normal blood pressure.

The importance of this WCRF finding is that the same factors that cause body fatness are the same factors that would increase the risk of cancers. Cancers and cardiovascular diseases are the top two causes of human death in the United States.

According to the Centers for Disease Control (CDC), *35% of the American population are obese and over 60% of Americans are considered overweight in 2010.*[2] That is a very significant jump from 15.1% being obese and 30% being overweight in 1980. Very alarmingly, over 17% of teenagers in the United States are considered obese. The big, fat problem of Americans has clearly become an obesity epidemic.

Managing a proper weight is the best way to maintain health and reduce the risk of major ailments and various disorders.

4.2 Understand the Basics of Weight Loss

4.2.1 It's Your Own Hormones

Many people work hard to lose weight by changing their diet habits and exercising regularly. But keeping weight off for the long term has been proven to be even harder. Study found that 83% of people regain most, if not all, of the weight that they've lost after two years[3]. Obesity is found to be a lot more resistant to conventional diet control. It becomes clear that eating the right foods, managing daily calories even with expert advice along the process, regular exercise, and strong willpower are not sufficient to solve the weight problem for the long haul.

One most important reason why managing weight is so hard and the weight-loss efforts of many people more often failed than succeeded is that they were fighting their own hormones.

The loss of body weight will trigger a hormonal change in our body that lowers metabolism. Leptin, which is a hormone produced by fat cells in our bodies that regulates metabolism and appetite, drops sharply with the loss of body fat. Columbia researchers[4] found that the level of the hormone leptin drops significantly when people lose 10% or more of their body weight. *The lower level of leptin will stay low even a year after the weight loss has occurred.* The drop of the leptin level to a certain threshold is sensed by the body and results in an increased urge to eat more and not feeling satisfied even after the stomach is full. The low leptin level also signals the brain to fight the loss of fat by slowing body metabolism. Slower metabolism results in less daily energy (calories) expenditure. The low level of leptin triggers the urge to eat and slows metabolism, and eventually dieters would not be able to fight their own biology and thus regain the weight. Leptin circulating in the blood is a key factor contributing to the difficulty of maintaining weight after weight loss.

Study also found that *leptin resistance* might be the leading cause of weight gain or difficulty losing weight in obese people. A high level of leptin is supposed to signal to the brain to reduce food intake. But this natural weight control mechanism in the body does not always work as expected. Researchers found that obese individuals have excessively high levels of leptin but continue to eat anyway. These people overfeed their bodies, but the perception from their brains is that they are still hungry. The long-term exposure to a high level of leptin in obese or overweight people creates leptin resistance, which reduces the sensitivity to the leptin signal and lessens the stimulation of the body's metabolism.

Leptin resistance leads to an increased appetite and the urge to continue eating. A dramatic drop of leptin after weight loss causes difficulty to maintain the weight.

A better way of trying to lose weight is trying not to gain it. People put on weight when they take in more calories than they burn. *Why do people continue eating even when their bodies no longer need the foods?* The sin of gluttony is not just a problem of overindulgence and failed willpower. Leptin resistance is one key cause of overeating even though the stomach is already full. The surge of chemical dopamine in the brain's pleasure center is another key factor. Researchers have observed the same spike of the chemical dopamine in the brain when obese individuals reacted to tasty foods and when drug addicts were tempted with drugs. Like drugs, sex, alcohol, and music, eating triggers a pleasurable feeling by overloading the brain with the happy chemical dopamine, which primes the brain to seek being high again. Foods that are tastier, with high sugar and high fat, incite stronger responses in the brain. There are evidences linking the behavior of overeating with the abundance of unhealthy foods that contain high fat and high sugar in the modern environment and the hijack of the brain by these kinds of foods.

Obesity is one of the greatest threats to our wellbeing and is a problem that researchers and society struggle to have a handle on. Solving the problem effectively for the long term requires not just diet control, exercise, and discipline.

The imbalance of appetite-regulating hormones makes weight maintenance and weight loss much difficult because they distort the normal appetite. Understanding the biology factors and how to restore the hormonal balance in the body is the key when a person wants to choose a diet or treatment that is truly effective for the long term. Instead of repeating the frustrated and futile "yo-yo" dieting of losing and regaining weight several times, dieters need to outsmart the hormones to have a long-term success in weight loss.

4.2.2 Ins and Outs of Calories

Ultimately it is the imbalance between the in calories from food intake and the out calories from energy expenditure that results in weight gain or loss. When the total calorie intake of the body is greater than the total calorie expenditure, people put on more weight even if they only eat healthy foods. When the total calorie intake is about balanced with the total calorie expenditure, people maintain stable weights. When the total calorie intake is lower than the total calorie used, people lose weight.

Hormones like leptin and dopamine in the brains affect the appetite and lead to overeating for people that causes higher calorie intake. Other factors like eating foods that are high in energy density or eating large portions of foods will increase the total calorie intake as well. While physical activities increase the total calorie expenditure.

PDA Weight Formula: The weight and calories relationship could be represented in the following formula:

Weight Change = (In Calories − Out Calories) x (Biology Factor)

In Calories is the total amount of calories that are taken in by your body through foods or drinks each day.

A large appetite, eating foods in large portions, eating when not hungry, and taking in energy-dense foods such as fast foods and sugary drinks are the main causes of high calorie intake. The imbalance of hormones like leptin and dopamine in the body plays a key role in causing the increased craving for foods for obese people.

Out Calories is the total amount of calories that your body burns each day. They include

1) Energy spent to maintain basic daily activities
2) Energy spent on extra physical activities, like sports, exercises, dancing, gardening, and yard work

Being physically active is the most direct way to increase out calories.

Biology Factor. It is as hard for a slim person to gain weight as for an obese person to lose weight. Individual genetic factor and body hormones determine how much the net positive calorie intake will be converted to body weight and how much body weight loss will be produced by the net negative calorie intake.

Daily Net Calorie Intake = In Calories — Out Calories

The same amounts of net calorie intake will be absorbed differently for different individuals because of biology factors.

Metabolism is the most important biological factor determining how much in calories will be burned out by the body and how much calories will be converted to fat. Obese people normally have low metabolism. There are many causes for a slow metabolism, including the hormones in our body. Stress and too little sleep will slow metabolism. A lower level of the hormone leptin when losing weight too fast will cause a slower metabolism. Lower levels of testosterone in our bodies when we age will cause slower metabolism.

Being physically active on a regular basis is the best way to boost metabolism.

Exercise Alone Is Not Enough. One of my friends Jane exercised vigorously and regularly but was puzzled about the little change in her body weight. Jane also had a very good appetite after exercise. The *PDA weight formula* could help her to explain the reason easily. The extra intake of calories with the big appetite after exercise has effectively offset the extra calories burned from the exercise. The net calorie intake (In Calories — Out Calories) is about balanced.

Eating Less Alone Is Not Enough. One of my friends John controlled the quantity of foods that he ate daily with discipline but found little change about his weight. John lives a sedentary life, without any physical exercise, and he ate foods with high energy sometimes. The *PDA weight formula* could help him to explain the reason as well. The calorie intake even with control of quantity is still no less than the calories burned to maintain his daily routines. The net calorie intake (In Calories — Out Calories) is about balanced.

After Weight Loss. After a dieter lost 10% of his weight, could he now eat or exercise less to maintain the lower weight level? The answer is no. The dieter who lost weight needs to continuously take in fewer calories or do extra exercise to burn more calories to maintain the lower weight. The *PDA weight formula* could explain the reason too. When a dieter lost weight, the lower level of the hormone leptin would signal the body to slow down its metabolism. A slower metabolism means more energy will be converted to fat (therefore less out calories). To maintain the lower weight, the man will need to do more activities to compensate for the lesser out calories. Or the man needs to lower his calorie intake to maintain the same net calorie intake.

4.2.3 Know Your Body Mass Index (BMI)

The body mass index (BMI) is a useful gauge of body fatness and is used to classify weight categories. Knowing your BMI will help you know exactly your current state of weight and know what your risk is for certain health conditions. Your BMI number will be very different if you are overweight by 10 pounds or 40 pounds.

An adult with a BMI between 18.5 and 25 is considered to have a normal weight. An adult with a BMI between 25 and 30 is considered overweight. An adult with a BMI over 30 is considered obese.

The body mass index (BMI) is a simple measure of height to weight ratio and is the most-often used method to classify the body. To find out your BMI, use the following formula:

BMI = Weight / (Height x Height)
(Weight in kilograms, height in meters)

The BMI for a man who is 5'11" (1.8m) and 180 lbs. (81.6 kg) is about 25.1. He is at the borderline of being overweight.

The BMI for a woman who is 5'5" (1.65m) and 150 lbs. (68.0 kg) is about 25. She is also at the borderline of being overweight.

There are many free Web sites available that let you calculate your BMI by simply entering your body weight and height.

4.3 PDA Strategies for Weight Management

Many dieters have tried diet plans or quick-fix programs to lose weight often in a short period of time. Most of these diet plans are not working for dieters because they only focus on foods and nutrients without the consideration of habits and biology factors that are equally important in daily food choices. The hormones in our body work against weight loss by increasing our craving for foods and lowering the body's metabolism rate when weight loss occurs. Suddenly including many new foods in your daily diet and giving up familiar foods that you used to eat is usually not natural to the body and causes major disruption both biologically and psychologically to the dieters. Following these diet plans, dieters have to move beyond their comfort zone to start to buy many new foods, learn how to cook them, adjust to the new tastes, and count calories or measure portion sizes. Most dieters do not have enough willpower to sustain the kind of unnatural change demanded by these diet plans. The fact is that long-term successful weight loss is not what most quick-fix programs can achieve.

PDA offers a unique new paradigm to manage weight. Instead of a diet program that dictates what you eat, PDA lets individual dieters proactively make small and gradual changes to their diet based on their own circumstance, own preference, and own pace that lead to habits and weight loss that would stick with them for life.

Based on the **PDA weight formula**, you could change one, two, or all three levers to achieve the goal of weight change that you desire.

Weight Change = (In Calories − Out Calories) x (Biology Factor)

PDA provides a set of strategies that are based on foods, activities, and biology, which are three key factors that strongly influence the body weight. No matter which strategy individual dieters choose to execute fully or partially, dieters are making positive progress toward the goal of healthy weight. PDA does not cause stress or guilt that is commonly associated with other diet programs. Over time the small changes lead to habits that stick with the dieters, and the approach will truly accomplish what many other diet recommendations had failed to do: successful long-term weight loss.

4.3.1 How to Reduce In Calories

For individuals who like to maintain the same level of daily activities, either because of a busy schedule or not being motivated enough to do more physical activities, limiting or reducing calorie intake wisely is the most direct way to maintain or lose weight based on the weight formula.

PDA provides five effective strategies that a person could apply to limit or reduce daily intake calories with immediate results.

1. **Avoid Energy-Dense Foods.** Energy density is the number of calories per weight of food. Energy-dense foods contain a lot of calories in a small amount of food. Most of these foods are processed foods, which contain substantial amounts of fat or sugar. High sugar and high fat energy-dense foods also trigger hormonal changes in the body. They stimulate appetite and slow metabolism.

   The worst energy-dense foods include highly processed fast foods, which are consumed frequently, like french fries, burgers, fried chickens, and milk shake. *One serving of large french fries could contain over 1,400 calories.* They are packed with calories, many unhealthy ingredients, and often come in large portions. Desserts, baked goods, and snacks are mostly high in energy density due to the substantial amounts of sugars and fats. Avoiding these kinds of foods is the most effective way to reduce calorie intake. It will also limit your risk to the harmful ingredients commonly associated with these foods.

2. **Avoid Sugary Drinks.** To burn 300 calories, an adult might need to run thirty minutes on a treadmill or do over one hour of brisk walking. A 12oz can of cola has about 140 calories, with 40 grams of sugar. Giving up sugary drinks like colas and sodas daily might be the low-hanging fruits for most people to reduce their calorie intakes.

The expert panel of the landmark World Cancer Research Fund (WCRF) report recommended total avoidance of sugary drinks if possible and that people should consume energy-dense foods sparingly. By reducing the risk of weight gain and body fat, the risk of some cancers is reduced.

3. **Eat the Best Foods.** Choosing the best foods in the five food groups is another effective way to reduce calories. Most of the best foods are naturally high in fiber and packed with healthy nutrients, are low in energy density, are less processed, and many of them are low glycemic index (GI) foods, which help to curb appetite and avoid overeating. Eating best foods offers a double bonus by leaving less room for unhealthy foods.

4. **Good Sleep and Less Stress.** Researchers found that not enough sleep and stress are directly linked to increased craving for foods and increased risk of body weight gain and diabetes.

Studies have shown clear evidence that not enough sleep for a few days causes a sharp drop in the level of the hormones leptin and ghrelin, which regulate appetite.[6] Lower levels of these hormones increase appetite and make you crave for more sugar and foods. Other than causing overeating, lack of sleep also causes slower metabolism, less insulin production by the pancreas, and higher blood sugar level.

Stress leads to releases of the hunger hormone ghrelin, which increases appetite and stimulates craving for energy-dense foods (high in calories). Stress also causes an increased level of the stress hormone cortisol, which increases appetite and cravings for salty and sweet foods. Cortisol can also cause hyperglycemia (high blood sugar), which could lead to diabetes.

Too little sleep and long-term stress induce excessive eating and more calorie intake. Getting enough sleep and managing stress is as important as a healthy diet and regular exercise. Getting more sleep is a good way to reduce calories.

5. **Control Your Eating.** Obese individuals are commonly found to have bigger appetites, eating more and eating larger portions than individuals who have regular body weight.

Adjusting daily eating tendency is a very important way to reduce calorie intake. Eating until you are full, eating when you are not hungry, ordering large portions of foods, ordering desserts after a meal, and eating in buffets will unnecessary increase your daily calorie intake.

4.3.2 How to Increase Out Calories

For individuals who prefer to keep their food intakes, because of either environmental limitations or the unwillingness to make adjustments, increasing physical activities is the single best alternative path to increase out calories, improve metabolism, and maintain a healthy weight.

Based on strong evidences that physical activity protects against cancer, weight gain, and obesity, the expert panel of the landmark World Cancer Research Fund (WCRF)[1] report recommended thirty to sixty minutes of moderate physical activity or thirty minutes or more of vigorous physical activities every day.

Physical activities help the body burn extra energy (calories) and lower the net intake of calories. Weight exercises, which increase muscle mass, will help body boost metabolism.

Researchers also found that physical activity offered a double bonus by restoring the hormonal balance in weight loss people, which will help them to have an improved metabolism. Because of leptin resistance, obese people have plenty of leptin yet remain obese. A moderate exercise of thirty minutes daily is found to trigger a metabolic change that can reverse leptin resistance. The cell becomes sensitive and responsive to leptin again.

Other than exercises like running, gym, and sports, physical activities might include walking, yard works, gardening, sex, and recreational activities like hiking, biking, and dancing.

4.3.3 How to Outsmart Your Hormones with Low Glycemic Index (GI) Foods

A hungry stomach increases hormones that make it hard for the body to resist overeating. When a dieter has lost weight too fast, a lower level of the hormone leptin in the body causes a slower metabolism to reverse the weight loss. A more effective way than skipping breakfasts or meals, or trying a quick-fix diet to lose weight initially, researchers found out that a diet with low glycemic index (GI) foods is the best among popular diets to manage a healthy weight with no negative side effect. A diet with low GI foods is similar to the Mediterranean diet and focuses on unprocessed foods like whole grains, nuts, vegetables, and fish.

In a study published in the *Journal of the American Medical Association*[5] in 2012, researchers compared three common diets: low-fat diet, low-carbohydrate diet, and low-glycemic-index diet. Energy expenditure for each diet was measured. Higher energy expenditure increases weight loss.

Individuals in the *low-fat diet* group ate mostly carbohydrates (60% percent of total calories from carbohydrates) and limited the amount of fats and the total calorie intake. The diet was found burning the lowest amount of energy, with some side effects such as increase of triglycerides and lowering of good cholesterol HDL.

Individuals in the *low-carbohydrate diet* group, which is modeled on the Atkins diet, ate a higher percentage of proteins and fats and limited their carbohydrate (less than 10% percent of total calories from carbohydrates) per day. The diet was found burning the highest amount of energy, 300 more calories than those in the low-fat diet. But the result also came with side effects, such as increase of the stress hormone cortisol.

Individuals in the *low-glycemic-index diet* group were found burning 150 more calories than those in the low-fat diet. The result came without any adverse effects.

Low-fat diet and low-carbohydrate diet came with long term downsides. Severely restricting or eliminating certain types of foods and nutrients over the long term required by these two approaches is hard to sustain for most dieters as studies have found.

Eating low glycemic index foods (GI) offers the best chance to long term weight loss with no negative side effect. It is also an effective way to outsmart the hormones. Low GI foods are slower in digestion and absorption. They are called slow carbs because the foods stay in the stomach longer and make the body feel full longer. Low GI foods help the body to be less likely to overeat by delaying the craving for foods and reducing the hormones that are associated with hunger. They also help to reduce insulin resistance by slowing the raising of blood-sugar level.

The *glycemic index (GI)* is a common way of classifying foods containing carbohydrates based on their potential to raise our blood-sugar levels. Foods from animals do not have GI scores. Foods are ranked based on a scale where food is assigned scores from 1 to 100.

Low GI foods = 0-55
Intermediate GI foods = 56-69
High GI foods = 70-100

Eating high GI foods (70 and above) increases blood-sugar levels to a high degree quickly, while eating low GI foods (55 and lower) raises blood-sugar levels slowly and over a longer period.

Examples of Low GI Foods in Different Food Groups

Vegetables	Kale, Broccoli, Bell Pepper, Cabbage, Spinach, Brussel Sprouts, Swiss Chard, Cauliflower, Tomatoes
Fruits	Apple, Kiwi, Cherries, Grapefruit, Strawberry, Grape, Orange
Grains	Amaranth, Barley, Brown Rice, Quinoa, Buckwheat
Protein	Red Beans, Kidney Beans, Lentils, Pinto Beans, Peanuts, Cashews
Other Foods	Low-Fat Yogurt, Chocolate Bar, Milk, Soy Milk

Examples of high GI foods include white breads, french fries, mashed potatoes, potatoes, cornflakes, cheerios, donuts, bagel, pumpkin, watermelon, and dates.

4.4 Summary

1. Convincing evidences in the landmark World Cancer Research Fund (WCRF) study link excessive body fatness to six cancers. Body fatness also increases the risk of heart diseases and many disorders. Two-thirds of adults are overweight and 35% are obese in the United States. Knowing your body mass index (BMI) will help you know exactly your current state of weight and know what your risk is for certain health conditions. There are many free Web sites available that let you calculate your BMI by simply entering your body weight and height.

2. PDA offers a unique truly effective new paradigm to manage or lose weight. Many diet plans and quick-fix weight-loss programs are not working for dieters in the long term because they don't take into consideration the habits and biology factors. Maintaining a healthy weight is not merely a problem of diet control and self-control. Weight change is a biological process. Hormones in our bodies fight against weight loss, and our natural mechanism regulating appetite and metabolism does not always work. Instead of a diet program that dictates what you eat and has low probability of working in the long term, PDA lets you proactively make small and gradual changes based on your own circumstance, own preference, and own pace that lead to habits and weight loss that would stick with you for life.

3. Weight change is ultimately determined by the net calories that the body takes in. The weight and calories relationship could be represented by the *PDA weight formula*:

    Weight Change = (In Calories − Out Calories) x (Biology Factor)

In Calories: This is the total amount of calories taken by your body through foods or drinks each day.

Out Calories: This is the total amount of calories that your body burns each day.

Biology Factor: Individual genetic factor and body hormones determine how much the net positive calorie intake will be converted to body weight and how much body weight loss will be produced by the net negative calorie intake.

People gain weight when the in calories are more than out calories. People lose weight when the out calories are more than in calories.

4. PDA provides practical and easy-to-follow strategies for you to proactively choose to start your journey to long-term healthy weight according to your own unique situation, your own preference, and your own pace and speed.

A. How to Reduce In Calories

If you are not ready to take on running or extra physical activities, limiting or reducing the calories wisely is the most direct way to maintain or lose weight. Any of the following strategies will help you immediately reduce the daily intake calories:

- Avoid energy-dense foods
- Avoid sugary drinks
- Eat the best foods
- Have a good sleep and less stress
- Control your eating

B. How to Outsmart Hormones with Low GI Foods

Do not skip breakfast and meal that will only increase hungry hormones in the body. Study found that eating low glycemic index (GI) foods is an effective way to outsmart hormones. Low GI foods are slower in digestion and absorption and help the body to be less likely to overeat by delaying the craving for foods and reducing the hormones that are associated with hungry appetite. Eating low GI foods also helps to reduce the insulin resistance by slowing the raising of blood-sugar level. List of low GI foods is available in Appendix C.

C. How to Increase Out Calories

If you do not like to make any compromise with your appetite, 30 minutes or more moderate physical activities a day is the best and only effective way to burn extra calories and helps the body to restore the hormone balance and improve metabolism.

5. Managing a healthy weight is the best way to stay healthy. It is a tough work for many people. But study found that even a small weight loss will improve one's blood-sugar level, blood pressure, and cholesterol level and lower the risk of heart disease and diabetes. It also improves moods, energy level, mobility, and overall quality of life.

CHAPTER 5

Choose Organic

According to the U.S. Department of Agriculture (USDA) report,[1] some of our most favorite and most nutritious fruits (like blueberries, strawberries, and apples) and vegetables (like kale, spinach, and bell peppers) are found to have the highest levels of pesticide residues, which could not be cleaned by washing or peeling.

Agricultural chemicals like pesticides and fertilizers are widely used in conventionally grown vegetables, fruits, and grains to increase yields and protect against pests. Choosing organic is the only way to avoid pesticide residues and other toxins when we eat vegetables, fruits, and grains.

Animals reared in industrial animal farms are fed regularly with antibiotics and synthetic growth hormones. They are fed with genetically modified (GM) grains that have pesticide residues. They are raised in unsanitary conditions, where they cannot move or interact freely. Choosing organic is the only way to limit exposure to the harmful toxins from meats and dairy.

According to the Grocery Manufacturers Association, *nearly 80% of the processed foods sold in the United States contain genetically modified (GM) ingredients*. Most Americans eat GM foods without knowing it. Conventional vegetable oils, including canola oils, are mostly from GM seeds. Soy milk, tofu, and soy by-products in chocolates, breads, and cereals are from genetically modified soy. Canadian honey contains one-third of its pollens from GM rapeseeds.

Corn is another heavily genetically modified food. Corn is everywhere in America, and high-fructose corn syrup (HFCS) is almost in all processed foods. Choosing organic is the only way if genetically modified (GM) food is a concern to you and your family.

There is still no consensus whether organic foods are more nutritious or tastier than conventionally grown varieties and whether chemical trace levels in conventional foods set by the Environmental Protection Agency (EPA) is safe enough for human consumption.

But there is no doubt that eating organic vegetables and fruits can limit regular exposure to pesticides and herbicides, and eating organic meats and dairy can limit exposure to antibiotics and growth hormones and reduce bad fat intake from conventional products. Study found that even a small exposure to pesticides is risky to unborn babies, infants, and children. Exposure to pesticides is linked to higher risk of attention deficit hyperactivity disorder (ADHD) for children.[2] Eating organic foods is essential to achieve the highest level of diet.

Organic farming is considered sustainable farming, which emphasizes on conservation of soil and water by using natural fertilizers, avoids the toxic and persistent pesticides and other chemicals, and raises animals in a more humane condition to decrease and prevent diseases.

5.1 Common Vegetables and Fruits

Not all conventionally grown vegetables have high pesticide-residue levels. The strategy to minimize exposure to unhealthy toxins is to avoid those conventionally grown common vegetables and fruits with the highest level of pesticide residues.

The saying "One apple a day keeps the doctor away" is quite true. Apple is a great food in the fruits group, with an abundance of polyphenols, which are heart healthy, along with many other healthy contents (like the soluble fiber pectin and vitamin C), and it is also an excellent low glycemic index (GI) food choice for losing weight.

However, apple is among the vegetables and fruits conventionally grown, carrying the most pesticide residues. The Pesticide Data Program[1] of the USDA found detectable pesticide residues in 90% or more of samples which include apples, celery, cherries, nectarines, peaches, and strawberries. Apple topped the list with 98% of more than 700 apple samples tested by USDA program found with pesticide residues. *Choosing organic is especially important when you eat vegetables and fruits that carry the highest levels of pesticide residues.*

Some vegetables and fruits conventionally grown have very low detectable pesticide residues according to the USDA report. Conventional onion was found to have less than 1% of detectable residues. The risk of exposure to pesticide residues is much limited when choosing to eat conventionally grown common vegetables and fruits with low pesticide residues.

In 2012, EPA announced that it would ban the future uses of pesticide azinphos-methyl (AZM) effective on September 30, 2012. AZM is an organophosphate insecticide that has been widely used on apples, blueberries, sweet and tart cherries, parsley, and pears. AZM is considered neurotoxic that has been banned in the European Union since 2006.

The Environmental Working Group (EWG),[6] a non-profit organization that publishes report on pesticide uses in the United States every year, recommended consumers to buy organic for the "Dirty Dozen" fruits and vegetables. EWG also provided a "Clean 15" list which includes vegetables and fruits that have the lowest amount of pesticide residues. The latest report of EWG is available at http://www.ewg.org/foodnews/summary.

5.2 Meats and Seafood

Not all meats are the same. Meats from organically raised animals are very different from meats from factory-farming animals. Nonorganic meats, dairy, and seafood are from animals injected with growth hormones and antibiotics and that grew in inhumane and unsanitary environments.

Other than antibiotics and hormones, meats and dairy from conventionally raised cows have high levels of pesticide residues because they are fed with conventionally grown, genetically modified grains.

The grass-fed organic beef has a lower total fat and is as lean as skinless chicken. It is the best source of the good fat conjugated linoleic acid (CLA), which was identified by research as a potent element against cancer and tumors. Grass-fed beef also contains higher important nutrients, like vitamin E (four times higher than grain-fed beef), omega-3 fatty acids, beta-carotene, vitamin B, and minerals.

The natural food for cow is grass. Cattle farmers feed them with GM corn and soybeans to fatten them up quicker. Conventionally raised beef has a much higher unhealthy saturated fat and therefore higher calories. The ratio of omega-6 to omega-3 of conventional beef is several times higher than the grass-fed beef. Omega-6 is pro-inflammatory. Eating foods with high ratio of omega-6 to omega-3 (ideal ratio is 1:1) causes an increased risk of inflammatory diseases, including cardiovascular diseases, diabetes, and cancer. Due to the unhealthy factory-farming environment, beef from grain-fed animals increases exposure to various harmful bacteria.

Similar to cattle factory farms, farmed fish are grown in densely packed pens or tanks or ocean lots with high levels of pesticides used to kill fish parasites, antibiotics, and contaminants like toxic dioxins, copper sulfate, mercury, and cancer-causing PCBs. Fish are fed with genetically modified corn and soy, antibiotics, and sulfa drugs to control infectious diseases. Farmed salmons are also fed with synthetic pigment to make the meat color pink instead of the unappealing grey color due to the lack of natural coloration from being in a farmed environment. The most common farm-raised fish include salmon, carp, tilapia, cod, catfish, bronzini, grouper, and trout.

Farm-raised fish have higher levels of pesticides, cancer-causing PCBs, dioxins, toxaphene and dieldrin, and mercury than wild fish. Studies have found that farmed fish provide lower beneficial omega-3 fats and higher omega-6 fats even though farmed fish contain much higher fat than wild fish. Farmed salmon have lower vitamin D than wild salmon.

Wild fish are also not free from toxins, depending on the environment that they inhabit. Many caught wild fish are detected with high levels of toxins. Study found that caught wild Chinook salmon from British Columbia have the highest levels of the cancer-linked toxin PBDE (polybrominated diphenyl ether), while Chinook from Alaska have the lowest.

We are what we eat. Eating wild caught fish provides more health benefits while limiting exposure to harmful pesticides, chemicals, and toxins associated with farmed-raised fish. Fish farms consist of offshore oceanic feedlots, causing harmful effects to wild fish and other marine life. The pesticides, bacteria, fish wastes, feeds, chemicals, and toxins associated with factory-farmed fish pollute waterways, lakes, and oceans.

5.3 Genetically Modified Foods

Genetically modified organisms (GMOs) are organisms created when a gene in a crop has been altered by bioengineering to enhance protection against plant diseases, enhance insect resistance, and herbicide resistance. For example, through modern biotechnology, proteins that are a natural defense against pests from a bacterium were transferred to crop plants to create plants that produce protein that is toxic when ingested by pests.

Genetically modified foods are certainly not all natural and considered nonorganic foods. The USDA organic rule prohibited any use of genetically engineered organisms in organic production.

Seventy-six percent of Americans believe that they have never eaten genetically modified foods, according to study. The fact is that nearly 80% of processed foods[3] on grocery shelves contain GMO ingredients because of the ubiquitous GMO soy and corn in packaged foods. High-fructose corn syrup is added to almost all processed foods. There is no FDA rule that requires GMO labeling in the United States, while over fifty other countries in the world including EU, Japan, and China mandate GMO labeling.

The most common GMO foods in the United States include soybeans, corn, rapeseeds, sugar beets, aspartame, rice, dairy, cotton, and Hawaiian papayas. North America is the largest producer of genetically modified foods in the world. Over 90% of soybeans[4] and 85% of corns[3] in the United States are genetically engineered for either herbicide resistance or pesticide resistance. Most farm animals and farm-raised fish are fed GMO corn or soy. Vegetables oils, including canola oil, are mostly from genetically modified seeds.

There are ongoing debates in America about the health risk to humans from GMO foods in the long term. Concerns include increased risk of allergies, lower immune system, contamination between GMO crops and non-GMO crops, and other unintended effects.

5.4 How to Read Organic Labels

The organic market is the fastest-growing segment of the food industry due to a growing demand. Understanding organic labels correctly is important for shoppers to make informed choices about organic foods.

FDA guidelines ask food manufacturers to voluntarily label foods to indicate whether foods have or have not been developed using bioengineering. The easiest way to avoid GMO foods is to buy certified-organic foods.

The green-and-white *USDA Organic Seal*[5] is a federal organic seal or label for certified USDA organic products, which are grown and processed according to strict USDA standards, meeting state or independent private organizations certification requirements. A USDA agent must inspect the farm fields and facilities annually to make sure all the federal rules and standards are met, including detailed records about soil and water testing, crop rotation, animal welfare, contamination, and prohibited synthetic substances.

There are two types of organic products allowed to wear the USDA Organic Seal:

- **100% Organic.** Organic products almost always wear the USDA Organic Seal. The food products must contain only organic ingredients, and they must have been grown and processed according to USDA standards, meeting state or independent private organizations requirements. Any genetically modified organism is prohibited in the growth and handling of organic foods.

- **Organic.** Organic products may wear the USDA Organic Seal. The product must contain at least 95% organic ingredients. The remaining 5% are nonorganic ingredients or synthetic substances that are allowed under USDA's National List of Allowed Substances.

There are also food products that are not allowed to carry the USDA Organic Seal but can carry the Organic label.

- **Made with Organic Ingredients.** The food products may contain between 70% to 94% organic ingredients. Up to 30% of the ingredients can be from nonorganic ingredients.
- **Contain Organic Ingredients.** The food products contain less than 70% organic ingredients. They can only list the organic ingredients on the ingredients panel of the food.

There are food products with the label Natural or Free Range. They are not considered as organic and are not allowed to carry the USDA Organic Seal or the Organic label.

5.5 Summary

1. "One **organic** apple a day keeps the doctor away" is more appropriate in the modern food environment. The average American is exposed to more than ten pesticide residues from foods, drinks, and water every day. Some of the healthiest vegetables (like spinach and kale) and fruits (like apples, blueberries, and strawberries) are also found to have the highest amount of pesticide residues. *Choosing organic is the best and only way to limit the risk of exposure to pesticides as well as antibiotics, hormones, toxins, and contaminants that are commonly associated with conventionally grown foods.* It is most important to choose organic when you eat vegetables and fruits that have

the highest level of pesticide residues. Nearly 80% of packaged foods in the United States contain GMO ingredients. Choosing organic is the only way to avoid any potential long-term risk that might be associated with eating GMO foods.

2. There are four organic labels allowed by the USDA National Organic Standards, based on the percentage of organic ingredients in the organic product: 100% Organic, Organic, Made with Organic Ingredients, Contains Organic Ingredients. Only two labels (100% Organic and Organic) may carry the USDA Organic Seal. Understanding different types of organic labels will help shoppers make informed decisions.

3. There is no doubt that choosing organic foods is the most ideal way to eat the best foods and is essential for an individual to achieve the advanced level of healthy diet. Choosing organic not only will protect you and your family from the toxins of traditional foods, it will also protect farm workers, the environment, and the animals.

CHAPTER 6

Conclusion

We are free to choose what we eat, how much we eat, how to eat, and our belief about food for whatever reasons. But we could not choose the consequences of what we eat to our body. According to the World Health Organization (WHO), unhealthy diets, physical inactivity, and smoking are responsible for about 80% of cardiovascular diseases, and at least 30% of cancers are due to dietary factors.[1] Cardiovascular diseases including heart disease and stroke are the number one cause of human death, and cancers are the number two leading cause of death in Western countries.

The fact supported by scientific research is that most people cannot just eat anything. Some foods are definitely bad for the body, giving people serious illnesses. Some foods have the opposite effects, being anti diseases. Some foods have very minimum nutrients and are even harmful to the body. Some foods are rich in nutrients that improve brain memory, are anti-inflammatory, and boost the overall wellbeing of our bodies. If we want a healthy body, we must make sure to have a diet that is in harmony with the basic universal law of health and is diverse and nutritional based on scientific evidences.

The foods available to humans are more abundant than any time in history. At the same time, our foods have an increased risk of harmful chemicals due to antibiotics, pesticides, growth hormones added to animal feeds, harmful additives and chemicals added to processed foods, unsafe environments (like polluted agricultural lands, rivers, lakes, and oceans), and the culture of unhealthy fast foods. On the positive side, we now have much more information than our ancestors had about what foods and nutrients are good or bad for our health.

Most of diet plans are not working for dieters in the long-term. Many dieters worked very hard to lose weight and found out that maintaining weight is even harder. Study found that over 83% of dieters regained most of the weight lost after two years. People are frustrated and dismayed, and obviously many approaches to diets are not so effective.

6.1 It's Never Too Late

David Murdock did not start his healthy diet routine until his sixties after both his mom and his wife died while they were only in their early forties. About 90 years old, Murdock still lives a robust life with a clear mind and an energy level higher than people several decades younger. He has been doing his own grocery shopping even though he is one of the richest men in America. The foods that he chose to eat that are the key to maintain his advanced level of health are available in the supermarkets that we all go to. He is still actively devoting his time and wealth to promote research and study about foods, nutrition, and disease prevention.

David Murdock is a great example. The story of David Murdock is that it is never too late to start for anyone. We could eat wisely to have an energetic and vibrant life that is free of major disease or minor ailment.

Wellbeing is a choice. It is not just about weight loss, it is about the absence of disease, being free of pains, having youthfulness and longevity, and your body being in a state filled with energy and vitality, where you are able to enjoy food and life to the fullest extent.

The power of eating the most nutritious foods can help you achieve the advanced level of wellbeing in the most efficient way.

6.2 Every Choice Has Big Impact

Brian was a senior consultant whom I used to work with for one of my business clients. We used to go out for lunches together quite often due to work relationship. He had worked in the U.S. military for some years. He was about forty years old. He liked to go to the gym in the morning and looked very strong with impressive physiques. He ate almost everything in lunches including some unhealthy choices such as sodas, fast foods, french fries, and potato chips. He told me that he loved to grill chickens and flank steaks at home. His wife and two kids loved the grilled foods. He believed that he had made the healthy choice since he always burned off the fats of the steaks over the frame of the grill so that the saturated fats would be totally gone. Sounds good?

Unfortunately, meats in high temperature are in the list of "most harmful foods to avoid." Researchers found that meats would form the cancer-causing chemical heterocyclic amine (HCA) when they are cooked at high temperatures (grilled or pan frying) above 300ºF or are cooked for long time. Amino acids and the protein creatine in meat form HCAs when meats are under high temperature. Skinless chicken breast, steak, pork, salmon with skin, and hamburger are the top five worst meats to grill that contain very high level of HCAs, according to research. *Skinless chicken breast is the worst with more than 10 times HCAs than steak when grilled.*[2] The more done and longer the time the meats are under high temperature, the higher amounts of HCAs would form. Medium rare beef is actually healthier than grilled chicken.

When meats are under direct flame and exposed to smoke or charring, another cancergen, polycyclic aromatic hydrocarbon (PAH), is formed.

Brian thought that he was making a safe choice with grilled chicken and beefs. But it turned out that he was wrong. Eating grilled chickens or burning the fats of steaks over flame is unhealthy for the body after all. After I had explained the research findings to Brian and sent him a few links, Brian had stopped using his home grill since. His family might have given up the enjoyment of grilled meats. But he had made a better trade-off because he knew that he would not like his family to eat to give themselves cancers.

When we went out lunches again, I noticed that Brian would hesitate with the menus if we went to restaurants with limited healthy foods. I was amazed with his new eating discipline. With what he had learned about the unhealthy foods now, it was no longer rational to just eat whatever he wanted. Obviously Brian had just acquired a new healthy habit that would stick with him and benefit him for a long time.

We make many small choices about food, snack, and drink daily. Every choice that we make will have a big impact on our wellbeing. With every bad food that we don't eat, we help our bodies to avoid its net negative effect. Eating the healthiest foods is the best path to live an active, satisfying, and vibrant life that will lead to longevity. Anyone could achieve the advanced level of diet, and it is never too late to start.

6.3 This Book Makes It Easy for You

The idea of the proactive diet approach (PDA) is that we need to change the way we think about how to eat. Eating cannot just focus on foods and nutrients and treat every food the same based on generalized recommendation. Not taking into consideration the human habits and biology factors that play an important role in people's daily eating is the main reason why many diet plans have not helped people improve the diet that they have intended to.

PDA shows people how to eat with the right knowledge. It is a comprehensive how-to-eat guide that has taken into consideration foods, habits, and biology factors. It provides four clear and effective strategies that common people can easily adopt in their own pace and enjoy; and with these, they'll be able to get more out of their eating every day, and no exceptional willpower is required.

- Eat the best foods
- Avoid the worst foods
- Achieve life-long healthy weight
- Choose organic

6.4 Improve Wellbeing

If your goal is to improve your overall wellbeing, eating is one thing that is within your control.

This book makes it easy for you to start your journey to advanced level of eating with practical and easy-to-follow strategies in chapter 2, chapter 3, and chapter 5. By making small and gradual changes in your own pace and speed, you make a choice for your wellbeing, and the changes will eventually become the diet habits that will stick with you for the long term.

Chapter 2: Eat the Best Foods. This chapter provides a list of best choices for each major food group (vegetables, fruits, grains, proteins, and other foods). Eating the best foods is the most direct and efficient way to improve your diet immediately. When you eat the healthiest foods that give your body the most nutrient benefits, you also leave less room for unhealthy foods. Most of the best foods are tasty and enjoyable. Adding one best food like walnut seems like a small change, but the impact is very big. This most nutrient-dense food provides many health-protective effects and benefits for your body.

Chapter 3: Avoid the Worst Foods. This chapter provides a list of the most harmful foods and a list of the most undesirable foods that people should avoid. Avoiding eating the most unhealthy and harmful foods that give ourselves minor ailments or major illness like heart disease, cancers, and diabetes is an essential and smart thing to do to live an active, satisfying, and vibrant life that is free of disease. Even small changes in your diet will have a significant impact to your overall health.

Chapter 5: Choose Organic. Some of the best fruits (like blueberries, apple, and strawberries) and best vegetables (like kale, spinach, and bell pepper) are among the most contaminated with pesticide if conventionally grown. Dieters should always go with organic because of the high level of pesticide residues in them. Choosing organic is the best and only way to limit the risk of exposure to pesticides as well as antibiotics, hormones, toxins, and contaminants that are commonly associated with conventionally grown foods.

6.5 Lifelong Healthy Weight

If your goal is to lose weight or maintain a healthy weight, you need to have a new perspective to have a successful long-term weight loss.

This book makes it easy for you to understand why maintaining a healthy weight is not merely a problem of diet control and self-control.

Chapter 4: Achieve Life-Long Healthy Weight. This chapter provides the latest scientific facts that overweight are more dangerous than people realize. Body fatness is found convincingly linked to six cancers more than any other lifestyle factors. PDA offers a unique new paradigm to manage a healthy weight for lifetime. Many diet plans are not working for dieters because they only focus on foods and nutrients without the consideration of habits and biology factors that are equally important in daily food choices. Instead of a diet program that dictates what you eat, PDA lets each dieter proactively make small and gradual changes based on the individual's own circumstance, own preference, and own pace that lead to habits that stick. PDA provides unique strategies to outsmart our own hormones that work against weight loss by increasing our craving for foods and lowering the body's metabolism rate when weight loss occurs.

We are free to choose what we eat, how much we eat, how to eat, and our belief about foods for whatever reasons. But we could not choose the consequence of what we eat to our body. Once you have built up plaque in your blood vessels due to long term unhealthy eating, it is much harder if not impossible to reverse the effect. How to eat right is a choice that will have a big impact on your wellbeing and happiness.

By reading this book, I genuinely hope that you have a clear picture about how to eat and enjoy food every day; and more importantly, you are able to help your family, your friends, your coworkers, and anyone you know to live a better life.

APPENDIX A

Best Foods for Each Food Group

List of Best Vegetables

Sweet Potato	Eating only one hundred grams (3.5 ounces) will provide 380% daily needs for vitamin A, 33% for vitamin C, 25% for manganese, 14% for potassium, and 13% for dietary fiber. It is a good source of other vitamins, like B6, pantothenic acid, and thiamin.
Kale	Eating only one hundred grams (3.5 ounces) will provide 272% of the daily requirement for vitamin A, 200% for vitamin C, a whopping 881% for vitamin K, and 33% for manganese.

Kale is very rich in plant-based omega-3s and is a good source of other nutrients, like calcium, magnesium, copper, potassium, and vitamin B6. |
| Broccoli | Eating only one hundred grams (3.5 ounces) will provide 149% of the daily requirement for vitamin C, 127% for vitamin K, 16% for folate, and 12% for vitamin A.

Broccoli has a very high amount of antioxidants. It contains the phytochemicals sulforaphane and indoles, which protect against cancers. |
| Spinach | It is one of the best sources for folate. Eating only one hundred grams (3.5 ounces) will provide 49% of the daily requirement for folate, 188% for vitamin A, 604% for vitamin K, 45% for manganese, 20% for magnesium, 16% for potassium, and 15% for iron. Spinach contains plenty of antioxidants, which few vegetables can match. |
| Seaweed | Seaweed is vegetable from the sea. Eating only one hundred grams (3.5 ounces) will provide 70% of the daily need for manganese, 49% for folate, 27% for magnesium, 15% for calcium, 14% for copper, and 12% for iron. |

Carrot	It has plenty of vitamin A and carotenoids, which few vegetables can match. Eating only one hundred grams (3.5 ounces) will provide 334% of the daily recommendation for vitamin A and an incredible amount of beta-carotene. It is a good source of potassium, vitamins B, C, K, and dietary fiber.
Red Bell Pepper	It is rich with antioxidants, like vitamin C, beta-carotene, and lycopene. Eating only one hundred grams (3.5 ounces) will provide 213% of the daily recommendation for vitamin C, 63% for vitamin A, 12% for vitamin B6, and 11% for folate.
Cabbage	It is rich with vitamin K and C. Eating only one hundred grams (3.5 ounces) will provide nearly 95% of the daily requirement for vitamin K, 61% of your vitamin C, and 11% for folate. One hundred grams of cabbage contain only 25 calories. Due to its low glycemic index (GI) profile, it is one of the ideal food choices for weight control.
Brussel Sprouts	Eating only one hundred grams (3.5 ounces) will provide 103% of the daily requirement for vitamin C, 175% for vitamin K, 15% for folate, and 16% for vitamin A.
Swiss Chard	Eating only one hundred grams (3.5 ounces) will provide nearly 122% of the daily requirement for vitamin A, a whopping 1,038% for vitamin K, 50% of your vitamin C, 20% for magnesium, and 18% for manganese. It contains incredible amount of lutein and zeaxanthin, which are carotenoids that protect the eyes.

List of Best Fruits

Blueberries	Blueberries and other berries like blackberries, cranberries, raspberries, and strawberries are great must-eat fruits. Blueberries have vast amount of health beneficial phytonutrients, which include anthocyanins antioxidant compounds that protect the plant against UV and are responsible for the bright colors of plants. Other than antioxidants, eating only one hundred grams (3.5 ounces) will provide nearly 16% of the daily requirement for vitamin C, 24% for vitamin K, 17% for manganese, and 10% for dietary fiber.
Kiwi	Studies show that eating kiwi daily is very heart healthy and helps to lower blood clot risk. The high level of the antioxidant lutein in kiwi is associated with eye health by lowering the risk of developing macular degeneration. Kiwi has almost twice the amount of vitamin C compared with orange. Eating only one hundred grams (3.5 ounces) will provide nearly 155% of the daily requirement for vitamin C, 50% of your vitamin K, and 12% for dietary fiber. Kiwi is also a good source of potassium, vitamin E, enzymes, folate, magnesium, and copper.
Guava	It has amazingly more than four times the amount of vitamin C compared with orange. Eating one hundred grams (3.5 ounces) will provide nearly 381% of the daily requirement for vitamin C, 22% for fiber, 12% for vitamin A, 12% for folate, and 12% for potassium.
Apple	The abundance of polyphenols in apples provides a special benefit to the cardiovascular system by reducing platelet in the arteries and lowering risk of many chronic heart problems. Other health benefits of apples include being anti-asthma, reduction in lung cancer risk, and weight control due to its low glycemic index (GI) profile. Apple is a good source of vitamin C and dietary fiber, including the soluble fiber pectin.

Avocado	It has the highest amount of heart-healthy monounsaturated fat among fruits. Monounsaturated fats provide protection against heart disease by lowering bad LDL cholesterol and raising good HDL cholesterol. Avocado has the highest amount of folate among fruits and has an incredible amount of dietary fiber. Eating one hundred grams (3.5 ounces) will provide nearly 27% of the daily requirement for dietary fiber, 17% for vitamin C, 35% for vitamin K, 20% for folate, 13% for vitamin B6, 14% for pantothenic acid, 14% for potassium, and 4% for protein.
Papaya	Eating one hundred grams (3.5 ounces) will provide 102% of the daily requirement for vitamin C, 19% for vitamin A, and 9% for folate. Papaya is also a good source of potassium, dietary fiber, vitamin E, and the enzyme papain, which helps digestion.

List of Best Grains

Oats	Eating only one hundred grams (3.5 ounces) will provide 42% of the daily recommendation for dietary fiber, 26% for iron and zinc, 31% for copper, 44% for magnesium, and an amazing 246% for manganese. Oats are also great sources for B vitamins like thiamin, folate, riboflavin, and pantothenic acid. Due to its low GI profile, it is one of the ideal food choices for weight control.
Quinoa	Quinoa protein is considered a complete protein source like meat or eggs, which has the adequate proportion of all nine of the essential amino acids. It contains all kinds of minerals like manganese, potassium, phosphorus, copper, iron, and magnesium which makes it an effective agent against cancer and heart disease, and it is anti-inflammatory. It is also a great source of vitamin B like folate, thiamin, riboflavin, B6 and vitamin E.
Amaranth	Amaranth protein is considered a complete protein source like meat or eggs, which has the adequate proportion of all nine of the essential amino acids. It is gluten free and has an exceptionally low glycemic index (GI).
Teff	Eating only one hundred grams (3.5 ounces) will provide 32% of the daily recommendation for dietary fiber, an amazing 462% for manganese (which is an essential mineral for bone health and builds blood and other connective tissues), and over 40% for iron, magnesium, phosphorus, and copper.
Kamut	Eating only one hundred grams (3.5 ounces) will provide an amazing 143% of the daily recommendation for manganese, 25% for iron and zinc, 26% for copper, 34% for magnesium, and 99% for selenium. It is also a great source of B vitamins like thiamin (39%), niacin (32%), vitamin B6, riboflavin, and pantothenic acid.

List of Best Proteins

Small Red Bean	Small red bean has an incredible amount of antioxidant content. Eating only one hundred grams (3.5 ounces) will provide an impressive 30% of the daily recommendation for dietary fiber and 16% for iron. It is a rich source of various minerals like magnesium, phosphorus, potassium, copper, manganese, and calcium. Red bean is also a good source of various vitamins like folate, thiamin, and vitamin B6. Other beans like red kidney bean and pinto bean have very similar health benefits profile like the small red bean.
Walnut	The nutrient content of walnut is so impressive that few other foods can match it. It has an incredibly amount of omega-3 content, which is protective to the heart and circulation. Eating one hundred grams (3.5 ounces) will provide 15.2 grams of protein, nearly 27% of the daily requirement for dietary fiber, an amazing 171% for manganese, 79% for copper, 40% for magnesium, 35% for phosphorus, 21% for zinc, 16% for iron, and 10% for calcium. It is an excellent source of vitamins like folate (25%), thiamin (23%), and vitamin B6 (27%).
Almond	Nearly 92% of almond fats are valuable, heart-healthy monounsaturated and polyunsaturated fats. Eating one hundred grams (3.5 ounces) will provide 21.2 grams of protein and provide nearly 49% of the daily requirement for dietary fiber, 114% for manganese, 50% for copper, 67% for magnesium, 48% for phosphorus, 26% for calcium, 21% for zinc, and 21% for iron. It is also an excellent source of the antioxidant *vitamin E (87%)* and other vitamins like riboflavin (60%), niacin (17%), thiamin (14%), and folate (12%).
Quinoa	Quinoa protein is considered a complete protein source like meat or eggs, which has the adequate proportion of all nine of the essential amino acids. It contains all kinds of minerals like manganese, potassium, phosphorus, copper, iron, magnesium which makes it an effective agent against cancer and heart disease, and it is anti-inflammatory. It is also a great source of vitamin B like folate, thiamin, riboflavin, B6 and vitamin E.

Salmon	Salmon contains an incredible amount of omega-3 fatty acids. Eating one hundred grams (3.5 ounces) will provide 22 grams of protein (44% of the daily requirement), provide nearly 59% of the daily requirement for selenium, 25% for phosphorus, 47% for vitamin B12, 40% for niacin, 32% for vitamin B6, and 23% for thiamin. The high amount of selenium in salmon is particularly important for reducing risk of joint inflammation and cardiovascular disease and aids in the prevention of cancers. Its being rich in minerals is also important for healthier skin, hair, and nails.
Anchovy	Anchovy contains an incredible amount of omega-3 fatty acids. Eating one hundred grams (3.5 ounces) will provide 28.9 grams of protein (58% of the daily requirement), provide 97% of the daily requirement for selenium, 100% for niacin, 26% for iron, 25% for phosphorus, 23% for calcium, 21% for riboflavin, and 11% for vitamin E.

List of Other Best Foods

Olive Oil	Seventy-six percent of fat in olive oil is monounsaturated fatty acids. Studies have shown that the very high content of monounsaturated fats in olive oil provide protection against heart disease. The plant phenols with potent antioxidant properties in olive oils improve blood circulation and protect blood vessels and cardiac tissues. The antioxidant and anti-inflammatory effects of olive oil have also provided prevention or reduction of the severity of arthritis and asthma. Extra-virgin olive oil (EVOO) that is cold-pressed is the best.
Yogurt	It has a high content of bone-healthy calcium. One cup of yogurt will provide 40-50% of most people's daily needs for calcium. What makes yogurt a superfood is that it is one of the best probiotic foods, containing healthy active bacteria with the power to protect the body in myriad ways.
Dark Chocolate	Plenty of flavonoids found in chocolates are found to be especially helpful in protecting the blood vessels and preventing high blood pressure through the antioxidant and anti-inflammatory properties of the said flavonoids.
Maple Syrup	Studies have found fifty-four amazing beneficial phenolic compounds in maple syrup, including five that are only unique in maple syrup. One ounce (28 grams) of maple syrup provides 46% of the daily requirement for manganese and 8% for zinc.
Red Wine	Studies have shown that drinking a moderate amount of red wine per week is particularly heart protective. Unique phytonutrients, particularly resveratrol, found in red wine have been widely studied and found to be especially helpful in protecting the blood vessels, reducing risk of inflammation and blood clotting, lowering bad LDL, and increasing good HDL.

List of Best Vegetables Based on Single Nutrient

Vegetables with the most potassium	Sweet potatoes, tomato paste, beet greens, white potatoes
Vegetables with the most antioxidants	Kale, Spinach, brussel sprout, beets, Red bell pepper
Vegetables with the most dietary fiber	Navy beans, kidney beans, black beans, pinto beans, lima beans, white beans, soybeans, split peas, chickpeas, black-eyed peas, lentils, artichokes
Vegetables with the most vitamin A	Sweet potatoes, pumpkin, carrots, spinach, kale, winter squash, red peppers, Chinese cabbage
Vegetables with the most vitamin C	Red and green peppers, sweet potatoes, kale, broccoli, brussels sprouts, cauliflower
Vegetables with the most folic acid	Seaweed, spinach, asparagus

APPENDIX B

Worst Foods to Avoid

List of Most Harmful Foods

Processed Meats	There is convincing evidence that processed meats increase the risk of colorectal cancer and raise the risk of heart disease and diabetes. Processed meats are mostly red meats that are preserved by addition of preservatives, salt, or by smoking or curing. They include bacon, sausage, ham, hot dogs, deli meat, pepperoni, and salami.
Starchy Foods in High Temperature	Starchy foods in high temperature produce a chemical called acrylamide. Potato chips and french fries are the top sources of acrylamide intake by the American population. Other top acrylamide foods include breakfast cereals, crackers, coffee, and toast.
Meats in High Temperature	Meats in high temperature produce the chemicals HCAs and PAHs, which are known carcinogens and found to increase cancer risks. Skinless chicken breast, steak, pork, salmon with skin, and hamburger are the top five worst meats to grill, which contain very high levels of HCAs. Skinless chicken breast is the worst that has more than ten times HCAs than steak.
Trans Fats	Trans fats are very harmful to the heart. FDA requires all food manufacturers to list trans fats amount in food labels. According to FDA, foods containing the most trans fats are microwave popcorn, cookies and cracker, bakeries, frozen pies and pizzas, breakfast cereals, margarines, and coffee creamers. FDA allows foods to be labeled "zero grams trans fats" even when they contain up 0.49 grams of trans fat per serving.

List of Undesirable Foods

Fast Foods	High amount of unhealthy fats and sodium, processed meats, chemicals, and cooking methods are what make these kinds of fast foods bad for the health. High calories lead to being overweight. High saturated fat intake has been linked to coronary heart disease and diabetes.
Refined Grains	Refined grains miss the health benefits provided by whole grains and cause spikes and crashes of blood sugar levels, which is not healthy to the heart and has an adverse effect on one's mood. Refined grains like white bread, regular white pasta, and white rice contain almost zero fiber and have lost most of their healthy nutrients like vitamins and minerals during the refining process, while whole grains reduce risk of diabetes and cardiovascular diseases by over 20%.
Sugar	The average American eats over 142 pounds of added sugar per year, according to USDA. This massive intake of sugar is what makes sugar detrimental to the health. It is a major factor in obesity and diabetes. One 12 oz can of cola contains about ten teaspoons (40 grams) of sugar.
Red Meats	Red meat from conventionally raised animals contains high amount of saturated fat and cholesterol. There are convincing evidences that eating red meat (beef, lamb, and pork) increases risk of cancers and heart diseases. The American Institute for Cancer Research recommends limiting intake of red meat to no more than eighteen ounces per week. Cancer risk rises when the amount of red meat consumed is beyond this amount.

APPENDIX C

Low Glycemic Index (GI) Foods

Examples of Low GI Foods in Different Food Groups

Vegetables	Kale, Broccoli, Bell Pepper, Cabbage, Spinach, Brussel Sprouts, Swiss Chard, Cauliflower, Tomatoes
Fruits	Apple, Kiwi, Cherries, Grapefruit, Strawberry, Grape, Orange
Grains	Amaranth, Barley, Brown Rice, Quinoa, Buckwheat
Protein	Red Beans, Kidney Beans, Lentils, Pinto Beans, Peanuts, Cashews
Other Foods	Low-Fat Yogurt, Chocolate Bar, Milk, Soy Milk

Examples of high GI foods include white breads, french fries, mashed potatoes, potatoes, cornflakes, cheerios, donuts, bagel, pumpkin, watermelon, and dates.

APPENDIX D

Glossary

acrylamide Starchy foods in high temperature produce a chemical called acrylamide. High acrylamide intake is linked to cancer in animal and human study.

antioxidants Chemical substances that inhibit oxidation by cleaning up the free radicals. Free radicals are by-products that the body makes during metabolism. They cause diseases by triggering chain reactions that damage body cells and are associated with chronic human diseases. Vitamin E is such a substance.

cardiovascular diseases Diseases that are related to the heart and blood vessels. When a blood clot forms due to plaque buildup in artery walls, it causes a heart attack or stroke. Cardiovascular diseases are the number one cause of human death in the world.

BMI The body mass index (BMI) is a simple measure of height-to-weight ratio and is the most-often used method to classify body weight categories. A higher BMI is linked to higher risk of heart diseases, diabetes, high blood pressure, and cancers.

diabetes Disorders wherein the body cannot regulate glucose (sugar) in the blood. *Type I diabetes* happen when the body has a problem producing the hormone insulin, which is responsible for taking glucose from the blood to body cells. This results in too much glucose in the blood. *Type II diabetes* happen when body resists insulin and results in too much glucose in the blood. High levels of glucose in the blood damage the cells and prevent them to function properly and can result in kidney and heart diseases. Type I diabetes are linked to generic and environmental factors that cause the body's immune system to attack the cells that produce the hormone insulin. Over 90% of diabetes are Type II diabetes, which are linked to being overweight.

dietary fiber Substance in vegetables and fruits that is important for the health of the digestive system and for lowering cholesterol. It is also good for binding and removing toxins from the colon and helps in blood-sugar regulation in diabetics.

dopamine Chemical in the brain that gives one pleasure or happy feeling when it is released. It plays a very big part in people's diets and other behaviors, like alcohol addiction, drugs, and sex.

essential amino acids To make all types of proteins that the body needs, our bodies require twenty different amino acids, and nine of them are called essential amino acids. They are considered essential because they must come from food and cannot be made by our bodies. Animals and plants are the two main sources for protein foods. Foods from animal sources like meat, poultry, seafood, and eggs are considered complete protein sources because they include all nine essential amino acids that our bodies need.

glycemic index Glycemic index (GI) is a common way of classifying foods containing carbs based on their potential to raise our blood-sugar level. Foods from animals do not have GI scores. Foods are ranked based on a scale where food is assigned scores from 1-100.

genetically modified organisms (GMOs) Organisms in which a gene in a crop has been altered by bioengineering to enhance protection against plant diseases, enhance insect resistance, and herbicide resistance. Genetically modified foods are considered nonorganic foods.

high density lipoprotein (HDL) Good cholesterol, which removes bad cholesterol from the bloodstream. Higher HDL levels in the blood lower the risk of heart disease. Lower HDL levels in the blood raise the risk of heart disease.

high blood pressure There is pressure against artery walls when the heart pumps blood through the body. High blood pressure is when the pressure against vessel walls stays high for a long period of time. High blood pressure damages the body and increases risk of heart attack and stroke.

inflammation The biological response of the body to fight infection and heal itself. Chronic inflammation is linked to many serious illnesses, like cancer and heart disease.

insulin Hormone produced by the pancreas, which is important for regulating carbohydrate and fat metabolism. When the body has a problem producing enough insulin or when the body resists insulin, this results in too much glucose in the blood and causes diabetes.

leptin Hormone that regulates appetite, metabolic rate, and fat storage in our bodies. When the level of leptin is low in the body, it signals the brain that fat storage is low and triggers the body to eat more and slow metabolism to conserve energy. High levels of leptin signals the brain to reduce food intake. The long-term exposure to a high level of leptin in obese or overweight people creates *leptin resistance*, which reduces the sensitivity to leptin signal and lessens the stimulation of the body's metabolism.

low density lipoprotein (LDL) Bad cholesterol that builds up plaques in the blood vessel walls. Plaques can narrow the vessel walls, causing coronary heart diseases.

low-carbohydrate diet Diet that involves eating higher percentages of proteins and fats and limiting carbohydrates to have a lesser percentage from the total calorie intake per day. The side effects of the diet include the increase of the stress hormone cortisol.

low-fat diet Diet that involves eating mostly carbohydrates and limited the amount of fats and total calorie intake. The diet burns lower amount of energy, with side effects, like increase of triglycerides and lowering of good cholesterol HDL.

low-glycemic-index diet Diet consists of low GI foods (GI score 55 and lower), which raise blood-sugar levels slowly and over a longer period.

metabolism Biological process that determines how much calorie intake will be burned out by the body and how much calories will be converted to fat. Obese people normally have low metabolism. There are many causes for slow metabolism, including hormones in our body. Stress and too little sleep will slow metabolism. Lower levels of the hormone leptin when losing weight too fast will cause a slower metabolism.

minerals Inorganic nutrients from food intakes that the body needs to maintain and develop normally. There are two types of minerals: macrominerals and trace minerals. Macrominerals are minerals that the body needs in large amounts, like calcium, potassium, phosphorus, and magnesium. Calcium is a good macromineral, which is important for healthy bones. Trace minerals are minerals that the body needs in tiny amounts, like iron, selenium, manganese, copper, and zinc.

omega-3 Fatty acids that are essential for our bodies to function normally. It helps to reduce inflammation, boosts the heart's health, and is protective against cancers and other conditions.

omega-6 Fatty acids that are essential for our bodies. It is pro-inflammatory. The ideal ratio of omega-6 to omega-3 is 1:1. Diet with too much of omega-6s and not enough of omega-3s contributes to many inflammation diseases.

phytonutrients Chemical components from plants that are vital nutrients for maintaining a healthy body, preventing diseases, keeping the body younger, and living longer. Beta-carotene and lycopene are powerful phytonutrients, which are important for the health of the body.

refined grains Grains like white bread, white rice, and white flour that have lost all their fiber and most of their nutrients like vitamin E and B (folate, thiamin, riboflavin, niacin) and minerals (iron, magnesium) during the refining process. Other than losing the most nutritious parts of the grain, refined grains are mostly starches, which are easily converted to blood sugar and send blood-sugar levels soaring.

trans fats Fats that are artificially produced through a hydrogenation process, wherein hydrogen is added to a natural vegetable oil under a heated condition to turn liquid oil into solid fat at room temperature to prolong the shelf life of the oil. Trans fats are inexpensive. Food manufacturers and restaurants use them to increase the shelf life of foods and enhance foods texture and stability. Over 80% of trans fats exist in processed foods.

vitamins Vital organic compounds from food intakes that the body needs to maintain and develop normally. There are thirteen kinds of vitamins—vitamin A, vitamin B (folate, riboflavin, thiamine, niacin, pantothenic acid, biotin B6 and B12), C, D, E, and K. Vitamin C is one of the most important vitamins; it fights infection, boosts the body's immune system, is critical for healthy growth of body tissues, and protects the skin.

whole grains Grains that retain the entire grain seed, which include the bran, germ, and the endosperm, while refined grain is mostly endosperm. Endosperm is energy dense and a good source of energy for our daily activities. But it is the nutrient-poor portion of the grain. Most of the nutrients of grains like fiber, vitamins, antioxidants, phytonutrients, and vitamins and minerals reside in the bran and germ components.

APPENDIX E

References

Chapter 1

1. ScienceDaily, *Dieting Does Not Work, Researchers Report, Apr. 5, 2007*. Available online at http://www.sciencedaily.com/releases/2007/04/070404162428.htm

2. G. J. Wang, A. Geliebter, N. D. Volkow, F. W. Telang, J. Logan, M. C. Jayne, K. Galanti, P. A. Selig, H. Han, W. Zhu, C. T. Wong, J. S. Fowler. *Enhanced Striatal Dopamine Release During Food Stimulation in Binge Eating Disorder. Obesity, 2011*. Available online at http://www.ncbi.nlm.nih.gov/pubmed/21350434

3. World Cancer Research Fund (WCRF), *Food, Nutrition, Physical Activity, and the Prevention of Cancer: a Global Perspective, 2012*. Available online at http://www.dietandcancerreport.org/cancer_resource_center/downloads/chapters/chapter_07.pdf

4. Centers for Disease Control (CDC), *Prevalence of Obesity in the United States, 2009-2010*. Available online at http://www.cdc.gov/nchs/data/databriefs/db82.pdf

5. U.S. Department of Agriculture (USDA), *MyPlate* is available online at http://www.choosemyplate.gov

6. U.S. Department of Agriculture (USDA), *National Nutrient Database for Standard Reference (Release 25)*. Available online at http://ndb.nal.usda.gov/ndb/foods/list

Chapter 2

1. F. Bruin, "*The Billionaire Who is Planning His 125th Birthday*", The New York Times, Mar. 30, 2011. Available online at http://www.nytimes.com/2011/03/06/magazine/06murdock-t.html?_r=0&adxnnl=1&ref=magazine&adxnnlx=1353534641-FVx0G38qvdzDB2 cwYUshdA

2. U.S. Department of Agriculture (USDA), *National Nutrient Database for Standard Reference (Release 25)*. Available online at http://ndb.nal.usda.gov/ndb/foods/list

3. S. Liu, J. E. Manson, M. J. Stampfer, F. B. Hu, E. Giovannucci, G. A. Colditz, C. H. Hennekens, and W. C. Willett. *A prospective study of whole-grain intake and risk of type 2 diabetes mellitus in US women*, American Journal of Public Health, 2000. Available online at http://www.ncbi.nlm.nih.gov/pmc/articles/PMC1447620/

4. T. T. Fung, F. B. Hu, M. A. Pereira, S. Liu, M. J. Stampfer, G. A. Colditz, and W. C. Willett. *Whole-grain intake and the risk of type 2 diabetes: a prospective study in men*, American Journal of Clinical Nutrition, 2002. Available online at http://ajcn.nutrition.org/content/76/3/535.full.pdf

5. ScienceDaily, *54 Beneficial Compounds Discovered in Pure Maple Syrup*, Mar. 30, 2011. Available online at http://www.sciencedaily.com/releases/2011/03/110330131316.htm

6. U.S. Food and Drug Administration (FDA), *Daily Reference Values, 2011*. Available online at http://www.fda.gov/Food/GuidanceComplianceRegulatory Information/GuidanceDocuments/FoodLabelingNutrition/Food LabelingGuide/ucm064928.htm

Chapter 3

1. World Cancer Research Fund (WCRF), *Food, Nutrition, Physical Activity, and the Prevention of Cancer: a Global Perspective, 2012*. Available online at http://www.dietandcancerreport.org/cancer_resource_center/downloads/chapters/chapter_07.pdf

2. Centers for Disease Control (CDC), *Prevalence of Obesity in the United States, 2009-2010*. Available online at http://www.cdc.gov/nchs/data/databriefs/db82.pdf

3. Centers for Disease Control (CDC), *National Diabetes Fact Sheet, 2011*. Available online at http://www.cdc.gov/diabetes/pubs/pdf/ndfs_2011.pdf

4. R. Micha, S. K. Wallace, D. Mozaffarian, *Red and Processed Meat Consumption and Risk of Incident Coronary Heart Disease, Stroke, and Diabetes Mellitus: A Systematic Review and Meta-Analysis. Circulation, May 17, 2010*. Available online at http://circ.ahajournals.org/content/121/21/2271.abstract?cited-by=yes&legid=circulationaha;121/21/2271

5. J. G. Hogervorst, L. J. Schouten, E. J. Konings, R. A. Goldbohm, P. A. Brandt, *A Prospective Study of Dietary Acrylamide Intake and the Risk*

of *Endometrial, Ovarian, and Breast Cancer. Cancer Epidemiol Biomarkers & Prevention, November 2007.* Available online at http://cebp.aacrjournals.org/content/16/11/2304.full

6. Environmental Protection Agency (EPA), *Consumer Fact Sheet on Acrylamide.* Available online at http://www.epa.gov/ogwdw/pdfs/factsheets/soc/acrylamide.pdf

7. The Cancer Project, *Chicken, Steak Top List of Five Most Dangerous Foods to Grill: Barbecuing Creates Carcinogenic Compound in Meats.* Available online at http://www.cancerproject.org/media/news/five_worst_foods_to_grill_1007.php

8. U.S. Food and Drug Administration (FDA), *Talking About Trans Fat: What You Need to Know.* Available online at http://www.fda.gov/food/resourcesforyou/consumers/ucm079609.htm

9. U.S. Department of Agriculture (USDA), *Dietary Assessment of Major Trends in U.S. Food Consumption, 1970-2005.* Available online at http://www.ers.usda.gov/media/210681/eib33_1_.pdf

10. American Institute for Cancer Research (AICR), *Recommendations for Cancer Prevention.* Available online at http://preventcancer.aicr.org/site/PageServer?pagename=recommendations_05_red_meat

11. A. Pan, Q. Sun, A. M. Bernstein, M. B. Schulze, J. E. Manson, M. J. Stampfer, W. C. Willett, F. B. Hu, *Red Meat Consumption and Mortality: Results From 2 Prospective Cohort Studies, Archives of Internal Medicine, 2012.* Available online at http://archinte.jamanetwork.com/article.aspx?articleid=1134845

Chapter 4

1. World Cancer Research Fund (WCRF), *Food, Nutrition, Physical Activity, and the Prevention of Cancer: a Global Perspective*, 2012. Available online at http://www.dietandcancerreport.org/cancer_resource_center/downloads/chapters/chapter_07.pdf

2. Centers for Disease Control (CDC), *Prevalence of Obesity in the United States, 2009-2010*. Available online at http://www.cdc.gov/nchs/data/databriefs/db82.pdf

3. ScienceDaily, *Dieting Does Not Work, Researchers Report, Apr. 5, 2007*. Available online at http://www.sciencedaily.com/releases/2007/04/070404162428.htm

4. M. Rosenbaum, E. M. Murphy, S. B. Heymsfield, D. E. Matthews, R. L. Leibel, *Low dose leptin administration reverses effects of sustained weight-reduction on energy expenditure and circulating concentrations of thyroid hormones, Journal of Clinical Endocrinology and Metabolism*, 2002. Available online at http://www.ncbi.nlm.nih.gov/pubmed/11994393

5. C. B. Ebbeling, J. F. Swain, H. A. Feldman, W. W. Wong, D. L. Hachey, E. Garcia-Lago, D. S. Ludwig, *Effects of Dietary Composition on Energy Expenditure During Weight-Loss Maintenance, Journal of the American Medical Association*, 2012. Available online at http://jama.jamanetwork.com/article.aspx?articleid=1199154

6. S. Taheri, L. Lin, D. Austin, T. Young, E. Mignot, *Short Sleep Duration Is Associated with Reduced Leptin, Elevated Ghrelin, and Increased Body Mass Index, Public Library of Science, Dec. 6, 2004*. Available online at http://www.plosmedicine.org/article/info:doi/10.1371/journal.pmed.0010062

Chapter 5

1. U.S. Department of Agriculture (USDA) *Pesticide Data Program*. Available online at http://www.ams.usda.gov/AMSv1.0/getfile?dDocName=STELDEV3003674

2. M. F. Bouchard, D. C. Bellinger, R. O. Wright, M. G. Weisskopf, *Attention-Deficit/Hyperactivity Disorder and Urinary Metabolites of Organophosphate Pesticides, Pediatrics, 2010*. Available online at http://pediatrics.aappublications.org/content/early/2010/05/17/peds.2009-3058.abstract

3. Center for Food Safety, *Genetically Engineered Crops*. Available online at http://www.centerforfoodsafety.org/campaign/genetically-engineered-food/crops

4. CBS News, *Figuring Out What's in Your Food, Oct. 12, 2012*. Available online at http://www.cbsnews.com/8301-18563_162-4086518.html

5. U.S. Department of Agriculture (USDA), *National Organic Program.* Available online at http://www.ams.usda.gov/AMSv1.0/ams.fetchTemplateData.do?&template=TemplateA&navID=NationalOrganicProgram&leftNav=NationalOrganicProgram&page=NOPOrganicLabeling

6. The Environmental Working Group (EWG). Available online at http://www.ewg.org/foodnews/summary/

Chapter 6

1. World Health Organization (WHO), *Cardiovascular Diseases Fact*. Available online at http://www.who.int/mediacentre/factsheets/fs317/en/index.html. *Cancer Fact*. Available online at http://www.who.int/mediacentre/factsheets/fs297/en/

2. The Cancer Project, *Chicken, Steak Top List of Five Most Dangerous Foods to Grill: Barbecuing Creates Carcinogenic Compound in Meats*. Available online at http://www.cancerproject.org/media/news/five_worst_foods_to_grill_1007.php

APPENDIX F

Disclaimer

The content and information in this book is solely for informational purposes. IT IS NOT INTENDED TO PROVIDE MEDICAL OR NUTRITION OR DIET OR EXERCISE ADVICE. Please don't apply any information contained in this book without consulting with your doctor or a qualified professional. For anyone under the age of eighteen, please do not read this book without consulting your parents. Neither the author nor International United Business Inc. or the publisher takes responsibility for any consequences from any dietary application, new diet or exercise, medication, or treatment that results from reading the information in this book.

The author is not a medical doctor, health adviser, physical trainer, or certified nutrient expert. The above information is only my personal opinion.

ABOUT THE AUTHOR

Bin Ke is the president and founder of International United Business Inc., a company that provides consulting and IT architecture services to top Fortune 500 companies and federal government agencies for over 15 years. He has BS and MS degrees in electrical engineering. He has a strong expertise in analyzing, modeling, and developing effective solutions for the complex problems of clients.

Bin Ke lives in Northern Virginia and is an avid tennis player. He believes in living a healthy lifestyle and devotes his time to studying facts about food, health, relationship, happiness, and wellbeing. He hopes to identify effective life patterns that people could use to improve their life.